LONGEVITY HEALTH SCIENCES

The Phoenix Conference

ANNALS OF THE NEW YORK ACADEMY OF SCIENCES

Volume 1055

LONGEVITY HEALTH SCIENCES

The Phoenix Conference

Edited by Richard G. Cutler, S. Mitchell Harman, Chris Heward, and Mike Gibbons

The New York Academy of Sciences
New York, New York
2005

Library of Congress Cataloging-in-Publication Data

Phoenix Conference on Longevity Health Science (2003 : Scottsdale, Ariz.)
  Longevity health sciences : the Phoenix conference / edited by Richard G. Cutler ... [et al.].
      p. ; cm. — (Annals of the New York Academy of Sciences ; 1055)
  "Phoenix Conference on Longevity Health Science held on December 11–14, 2003 in Scottsdale, Arizona"—Contents p.
  Includes bibliographical references and index.
  ISBN 1-57331-561-3 (cloth : alk. paper) -- ISBN 1-57331-562-1 (pbk. : alk. paper)
  1. Longevity—Congresses. 2. Aging—Congresses.
  [DNLM: 1. Longevity—physiology—Congresses. 2. Aging—physiology—Congresses. 3. Longevity—genetics—Congresses. 4. Oxidative Stress—physiology—Congresses. WT 116 P574L 2005] I. Cutler, Richard G. II. Title. III. Series.
  Q11.N5 vol. 1055
  [QP85]
  500 s—dc22
  [613   2005029224

GYAT/PCP
Printed in the United States of America
ISBN 1-57331-561-3 (cloth)
ISBN 1-57331-562-1 (paper)
ISSN 0077-8923

ANNALS OF THE NEW YORK ACADEMY OF SCIENCES

Volume 1055
December 2005

LONGEVITY HEALTH SCIENCES
The Phoenix Conference

Editors
RICHARD G. CUTLER, S. MITCHELL HARMAN, CHRIS HEWARD,
AND MIKE GIBBONS

This volume presents a selection of the proceedings of **The Phoenix Conference on Longevity Health Sciences** held on December 11–14, 2003 in Scottsdale, Arizona.

CONTENTS

Preface. *By* RICHARD G. CUTLER   ix

The Involvement of Thioredoxin and Thioredoxin Binding Protein-2 on
   Cellular Proliferation and Aging Process. *By* TORU YOSHIDA, HAJIME
   NAKAMURA, HIROSHI MASUTANI, AND JUNJI YODOI   1

The Different Paths to Age One Hundred. *By* THOMAS PERLS   13

Genetic Engineering of Mice to Test the Oxidative Damage Theory of Aging.
   By GEORGE M. MARTIN   26

Aging and Genome Maintenance. *By* JAN VIJG, RITA A. BUSUTTIL, RUMANA
   BAHAR, AND MARTIJN E.T. DOLLÉ   35

The Use of Genetic SNPs as New Diagnostic Markers in Preventive Medicine.
   By CHARLES R. CANTOR   48

Longevity Determinant Genes: What is the Evidence? What's the Importance?
   Panel Discussion. *By* RICHARD CUTLER, *Moderator*: L.P. GUARANTE,
   THOMAS W. KENSLER, FRED NAFTOLIN, DEAN P. JONES, CHARLES R.
   CANTOR, GEORGE M. MARTIN, *Panelists*   58

Decoding the Pyramid: A Systems-Biological Approach to Nutrigenomics. *By*
   JIM KAPUT   64

Effects of Testosterone on Cognitive and Brain Aging in Elderly Men. *By*
   SCOTT D. MOFFAT   80

Oxidative Stress Profiling: Part I. Its Potential Importance in the
   Optimization of Human Health. *By* RICHARD G. CUTLER   93

Oxidative Stress Profiling: Part II. Theory, Technology, and Practice. *By* RICHARD G. CUTLER, JOHN PLUMMER, KAJAL CHOWDHURY, AND CHRISTOPHER HEWARD 136

Controversies in Dyslipidemias: Atheroprevention in Diabetes and Insulin Resistance. *By* ELIOT A. BRINTON 159

Dietary Fat and Health: The Evidence and the Politics of Prevention: Careful Use of Dietary Fats Can Improve Life and Prevent Disease. *By* WILLIAM E.M. LANDS 179

Physical Activity and Aging. *By* KERRY J. STEWART 193

Would Doubling the Human Life Span Be a Net Positive or Negative for Us, Either as Individuals or as a Society? Point–Counterpoint. *By* GREGORY B. STOCK AND DANIEL CALLAHAN 207

Abstracts

Regulatory Mechanisms Controlling Gene Expression Mediated by the Antioxidant Response Element. *By* THOMAS W. KENSLER 219

Targeting Redox Signaling Pathways for Anti-Inflammatory and Anti-Ischemic Drug Discovery. *By* GUY MILLER 220

Mitochondrial Thioredoxin: Critical Protection for the Redox Throttle of Life. *By* DEAN P. JONES 221

Regulation of Aging by SIR2. *By* LEONARD P. GUARANTE 222

Androgens in the Aging Man. *By* WILLIAM J. BREMNER 223

Potential Adverse Effects of Administering Testosterone to Elderly Men. *By* PETER J. SNYDER 224

Testosterone in Women. *By* ADRIAN S. DOBS 225

Estrogen: Metabolism, Actions and Effects. *By* JAMES W. SIMPKINS 226

Estrogen and the Heart: Choices for Prevention of Coronary Vascular Disease. *By* DAVID M. HERRINGTON 227

Estrogen, Cognition, and Dementia. *By* SANJAY ASTHANA 228

Use of Growth Hormone for Prevention of Effects of Aging. *By* S. MITCHELL HARMAN 229

Cardiovascular Risk Assessment. *By* HARVEY S. HECHT 231

Index of Contributors 233

Financial contributions were made by:

- AURORA FOUNDATION
- EXETER LIFE SCIENCES
- INTERNATIONAL SOCIETY FOR HEALTHY AGING RESEARCH (ISHARE)
- KRONOS LABORATORY RESEARCH INSTITUTE
- OXIDATIVE STRESS AND AGING ASSOCIATION (O2SA)

Preface

RICHARD G. CUTLER

Kronos Science Laboratory, Phoenix, Arizona 85016, USA

This volume contains the papers and abstracts presented at the First Annual Phoenix Conference on Longevity Health Sciences held at the Westin Kirland Resort and Spa in Scottsdale, Arizona on December 11–14, 2003. This meeting represented the first major conference designed to accelerate the rate of basic discovery and practical applications in the new field of Longevity Health Sciences and Medicine.

The conference was organized and supported by three members of the Kronos Group: S. Mitchell Harman of the Kronos Longevity Research Institute (KLRI), Richard G. Cutler of the Kronos Science Laboratoty and Oxidative Stress and Aging Association (O2SA), and Mike Gibbons of the International Society for Healthy Aging Research and Education (ISHARE).

At this first-of-its-kind conference, the Phoenix Conference proudly introduced and honored the extraordinary faculty that was assembled. These remarkable groups of individuals were drawn from a spectrum of different fields of specialization whose research has already shaped and will continue to shape how we live and work in the future. It was our aim that this conference and those yet to be held will lead the way in informing both lay and professional communities regarding this age of innovation in gerontology and optimal health achievement.

Even in economically tight times, the demand for effective treatments and innovation in the field of Longevity Sciences continues to rise, and perhaps never has been so important. Globally and domestically, in our communities and in all parts of our society, the creative passion for discovery aimed at improving health and the quality of life is as robust as ever. The purpose of this conference and of this volume is to achieve that goal. It is clear from the reports herein that the goal was indeed met

The research and clinical issues presented at this conference focused on three areas of Longevity Health Sciences, with one day provided to each area. The first area examined the role oxidative stress–related damage may have in causing age-related illness as well as the present and possible dietary, pharmaceutical, and exercise-related therapies that might reduce its adverse

Address for correspondence: Richard Cutler, Ph.D., Kronos Science Laboratory, 2222 E. Highland Avenue, Suite 220, Phoenix AZ 85016. Voice: 606-778-7488.
Richard.Cutler@KronosLaboratory.com

Ann. N.Y. Acad. Sci. 1055: ix–x (2005). © 2005 New York Academy of Sciences.
doi: 10.1196/annals.1323.034

health effects. The second area examined the real risks and benefits of hormone replacement therapy, while the last part examined practical measures that can be taken now to improve and optimize health and longevity for ourselves and our patients.

Many individuals were responsible for the planning and organization of this first Phoenix Conference on Longevity Health Sciences as well as in the publication of the proceedings and we would like to thank them all. We would like to especially thank Dr. Henry Rodriguez of the Biotechnology Division, NIST, and many of the staff members of KLRI, O2SA and ISHARE. Our appreciation is also extended to Caroline Essavi, for her invaluable contribution in helping in the book's production, and to the editorial staff of the *Annals* of the New York Academy of Sciences, who saw this volume through the press.

The Involvement of Thioredoxin and Thioredoxin Binding Protein-2 on Cellular Proliferation and Aging Process

TORU YOSHIDA,[a] HAJIME NAKAMURA,[b] HIROSHI MASUTANI,[a] AND JUNJI YODOI[a,b]

[a]*Department of Biological Responses, Institute for Virus Research, Kyoto University, Sakyo-ku, Kyoto, Japan 606-8507*

[b]*Thioredoxin Project, Translational Research Center, Kyoto University Hospital, Kyoto, Japan 606-8507*

ABSTRACT: Recent reports on aging have revealed that many genetic loci affecting life span are closely linked to the machinery either producing or defending oxidative stress. Protective mechanisms against oxidative stress are thus important in countering the aging process. Thioredoxin (TRX) is a small thiol-mediated protein with a redox-active disulfide/dithiol within the conserved active site. TRX transgenic mice are more resistant than control mice to a variety of oxidative stresses including infection and inflammation. Moreover, we observed that the median life span of TRX tg mice was extended up to 135% compared to that of controls. TRX binding protein-2 (TBP-2), which is identical to vitamin D3 upregulated protein 1 (VDUP1), was identified as a binding molecule to TRX, and a negative regulator of TRX function. The expression of TBP-2/VDUP1 is frequently lost in tumor tissue and cell lines, and ectopic expression of TBP-2/VDUP1 suppresses cellular proliferation along with cell cycle arrest at the G_1 phase. These findings suggest that TRX and TBP-2/VDUP1 are involved not only in cytoprotective functions against oxidative stress, but also in the regulation of cellular proliferation and the aging process.

KEYWORDS: thioredoxin; thioredoxin binding protein-2; aging; cellular proliferation; redox regulation

Address for correspondence: Dr. Junji Yodoi, Department of Biological Responses, Institute for Virus Research, Kyoto University, 53 Shogoin Kawahara-cho, Sakyo-ku, Kyoto, Japan 606-8507. Voice: +81-75-751-4024; fax: +81-75-761-5766.
 yodoi@virus.kyoto-u.ac.jp

Ann. N.Y. Acad. Sci. 1055: 1–12 (2005). © 2005 New York Academy of Sciences.
doi: 10.1196/annals.1323.002

TABLE 1. Life-span mutants in experimental model organisms

Loci	Species	Life Span	Putative Protein Function	Ref.
sir-2	S. cerevisiae	−50%*	NAD-dependent deacetylase	58
gas-1	C. elegans	−25%	electron transport complex I	7
mev-1	C. elegans	−30%	electron transport complex II	6
top3β	mouse	−35%*	DNA topoisomerase β	59
ttd	mouse	−50%*	nucleotide excision repair	47
[p53]	mouse	−65%***	tumor suppressor	50
msra	mouse	−40%*	methionine sulfoxide reductase	15
ku86	mouse	−61%*	double-strand-break DNA repair	48
terc	mouse	ND	teromerase	51
mth	D. melanogaster	35%*	G protein–coupling receptor	60
indy	D. melanogaster	+50%***	sodium dicarboxylate co-transporter	61
[sod]	D. melanogaster	+48%	superoxide dismutase	62
[sod/cat]	D. melanogaster	+30	superoxide dismutase/catalase	10
[msra]	D. melanogaster	+70%	methionine sulfoxide reductase	11
age-1	C. elegans	+110%***	PI3K p110 subunit	63
daf-2	C. elegans	+100%	insulin-like/IGF-I receptor	64
daf-16	C. elegans	ND	forkhead transcription factor	65
clk-1	C. elegans	+175%*	co-enzyme Q synthesis	8
isp-1	C. elegans	+62%	electron transport complex III	5
inr	D. melanogaster	+85%	insulin-like receptor	66
chico	D. melanogaster	+48%**	insulin receptor substrate	67
p66shc	mouse	+30%*	tyrosine receptor adapter	13
ghr	mouse	+55%*	growth hormone receptor	68
inr	mouse	+18%*	insulin receptor	69
ig1r	mouse	+33%*	IGF-1 receptor	70
[trx]	mouse	+35%**	thioredoxin	28

[a]When life span varies among sex, longest life spans are adopted. The listed life spans are average(*), median(**), or maximum(***), depending on the source, and no symbol imdicates that it was not described in the source. Life spans of hetrozygous mutants are indicated in case lethal phenotypes were observed in homozygous mutants.

NOTE: Brackets indicate transgenic strain or augmented expressions of the loci; ND, not described in detail or ineffective effect by locus alone.

LIFE-SPAN MUTANTS AND OXIDATIVE STRESS

There is accumulating evidence that many genetic loci affect life span, and these have been isolated from various experimental model organisms and categorized into components of either the insulin signaling pathway or energy production machinery (TABLE 1).It should be noted that life-span mutants simultaneously demonstrated strong resistance to reactive oxygen species

(ROS) and other free radical species. For instance, *age-1* and *daf-2* mutations in *C. elegans* showed strong resistance to oxidative stress[1-3] and increased mitochondrial Mn-SOD activities.[4] Moreover, many extended and reduced life-span mutation genes have been found to be components of the mitochondrial electron transport system, such as *clk-1* (CoQ enzyme), *isp-1* (complex III), *gas-1* (complex I), and *mev-1* (complex II).[5-8]

Methuselah (*mth*) was first isolated as an extended life-span mutant in *D. melanogaster* and was found to show strong resistance to paraquat-induced oxidative stress.[9] Transgenic fruit flies showed significant extensions of life span in several experiments introducing SOD and catalase,[10] msra,[11] and human SOD-1 into locomotor neurons.[12] At least two studies of knockout mice suggested evidence of a direct connection between oxidative stress and life span. One study showed that p66[shc−/−] mice had significantly extended life spans and enhanced resistance to paraquat-induced oxidative stress.[13] The ablation of p66[shc−/−] also enhanced cellular resistance to plasma LDL oxidation, arterial oxidation epitopes, and early atherogenic lesions.[14] Another study showed that methionine sulfoxide reductase A knockout (msra[−/−]) mice had shorter life spans and had higher sensitivity towards oxidative stress than controls.[15]

As for the biological function of *msra*, it has been shown to catalyze the reduction of oxidized methionine in protein by converting methionine sulfoxide to methionine. The catalytic enzyme reaction is completely dependent on the TRX redox system. TRX can serve as an electron donor in order to reduce the oxidized form of msra, and therefore the effective reaction of msra is closely associated with TRX, TRX reductase and NADPH. Meanwhile, Ruan *et al.* recently reported that *msra* transgenic animals showed significant resistance to paraquat-induced oxidative stress as well as extended life spans.[11] It will be intriguing to study further the effects of possible interactions between msra and TRX on the role of *msra*-mediated life-span extension.

THIOREDOXIN

Human TRX has been cloned as an adult T cell leukemia–derived factor (ADF), produced by human T cell leukemia virus I–transformed T cells,[16,17] or as an interleukin 1-like autocrine growth factor from Epstein-Barr virus-transformed cells.[8] TRX is a 12kDa thiol-mediated protein with a redox-active disulfide/dithiol within the conserved active-site sequence Cys-Gly-Pro-Cys. Reduced TRX catalyzes the reduction of disulfide bonds in many proteins, and oxidized TRX is reversibly reduced by the action of TRX reductase and NADPH[19] (Fig. 1).

The TRX system (TRX, TRX reductase, and NAPDH) is widely conserved from prokaryotes to eukaryotes. TRX was originally identified in *Escherichia*

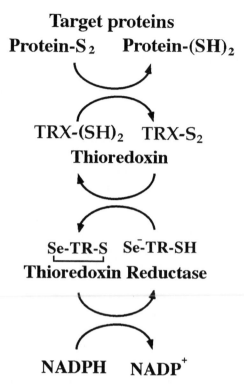

Target proteins

Protein-S$_2$ Protein-(SH)$_2$

TRX-(SH)$_2$ TRX-S$_2$
Thioredoxin

Se-TR-S   Se$^-$-TR-SH
Thioredoxin Reductase

NADPH   NADP$^+$

FIGURE 1. The thioredoxin system. TRX exists in either a reduced form containing two thiol groups or an oxidized form containing a disulfide bond. Oxidized TRX is reduced by TRX reductase and NADPH. The reduced form of TRX can reduce disulfide bonds of target proteins in association with NADPH and TRX reductase (TR). SeS: selenocysteine.

coli as an electron donor for ribonucleotide reductase, an essential enzyme in the production of deoxyribonucleotides for DNA synthesis. Disruption of the TRX gene significantly prolonged the cell cycle in *Saccharomyces cerevisiae.* [20] The TRX homologue gene was identified in *Drosophila melanogaster* and is required for female meiosis and early embryonic development.[21] Moreover, TRX knockout mice were found to be embryonically lethal.[22] Human TRX plays a key role in the redox regulation of signal transduction. TRX enhances the DNA binding of transcriptional factors such as AP-1 and p53.[23, 24] In addition, TRX regulates signal transduction for apoptosis. TRX is reported to be a negative regulator of apoptosis signal regulating kinase-1 (ASK-1). When TRX is oxidized by ROS, the binding of TRX and ASK-1 is disrupted and ASK-1 is activated to transduce apoptosis signals.[25] TRX also regulates tumor suppressor PTEN phosphatase, which regulates many cellular process through direct antagonism of PI3-kinase signaling.[26]

TRX-OVEREXPRESSING TRANSGENIC MICE

TRX has recently attracted much attention due to its strong anti-oxyradical quenching capabilities and other important biological functions related to the regulation of cellular redox state. We produced TRX-overexpressing transgenic (tg) mice, in which the human TRX gene was systemically expressed under the control of the actin promoter.[27] Focal cerebral ischemia is attenuated in these mice,[27] and they are more resistant to various inflammatory reactions and infections, such as influenza virus–induced pneumonia,[28] bleomycin-induced lung injury,[29] adriamycin-induced cardiotoxicity,[30] and cytokine-induced interstitial pneumonia.[29] These studies demonstrated that TRX may play an important role in the primary host defense against infection by modulating the ROS generation induced by influenza virus infection, and may regulate redox-dependent signal transduction in host defense responses. Elevated levels of TRX in the circulation of TRX tg mice also blocked chemotaxis induced by LPS or chemokines, showing the beneficial effects of acutely elevated TRX in inflammatory regions by suppressing neutrophil migration.[31] Physiologically, TRX has cytoprotective effects against oxidative stress by scavenging ROS by itself and/or together with peroxiredoxin. The bone marrow cells from TRX tg mice were more resistant to ultraviolet C–induced cytocide, and the survival ratio of colony-forming unit/macrophage (CFU-GM) after exposure increased compared to that of wild-type controls. Moreover, TRX tg mice had extended maximum life spans (22%) and median life spans (35%).[32] Telomerase activity in TRX tg mice from the spleen was also higher than in wild-type controls.[32] These reports demonstrated that TRX has shown not only redox regulation of the host defense mechanism, but also the direct influence of the TRX redox system on the generation of ROS, various stress-induced stimuli, and an animal's life span.

TRX FAMILY MOLECULES

Proteins similar to TRX, sharing the active-site sequence -Cys-Xxx-Yyy-Cys- are designated as members of TRX family (TABLE 2). TRX-2 is encoded as an 18kDa protein with a conserved TRX catalytic site, possesses a mitochondrial translocation signal, and is localized in mitochondria.[33,34] TRX-2 is expressed uniquely in mitochondria, where it regulates the mitochondrial redox state and plays an important role in cell proliferation. TRX-2-deficient cells fall into apoptosis via the mitochondria-mediated apoptosis signaling pathway.[35] TRX-2 was found to form a complex with cytochrome *c* localized in the mitochondrial matrix, and the release of cytochrome *c* from the mitochondria was significantly enhanced when expression of TRX-2 was inhibited. Overexpression of TRX-2 produced resistance to oxidant-induced apoptosis in human ostosarcoma cells, indicating a critical role for the protein

TABLE 2. TRX superfamily molecules

TRX Family Gene	kD	Localization	Active-site Sequence
Thioredoxin (TRX)	12	cytosol	-Cys-Gly-Pro-Cys-
Thioredoxin-2 (TRX-2)	12	Mt	-Cys-Gly-Pro-Cys-
TRX-related protein 32 (TRP32)		cytosol	-Cys-Gly-Pro-Cys-
Transmembrane TRX-related protein (TMX)	30	ER	-Cys-Pro-Ala-Cys-
Sperm-specific TRX-1 (SpTRX1)	53	fibrous sheath	-Cys-Gly-Pro-Cys-
Sperm-specific TRX-2 (SpTRX2)	67	fibrous sheath	-Cys-Gly-Pro-Cys-
Sperm-specific TRX3 (SpTRX3)	15	Golgi apparatus	-Cys-Gly-Pro-Cys-
Glutaredoxin (GRX)	12	cytosol	-Cys-Gly-Tyr-Cys-
Glutaredoxin-2 (GRX-2)	18	nucleus, Mt	-Cys-Ser-Tyr-Cys-
Nucleoredoxin	48	nucleus	-Cys-Pro-Pro-Cys-
Protein disulfide isomerase (PDI)	55	ER	$-[Cys-Gly-His-Cys]_2-$
Ca binding protein 1 (CaBP1)	49	ER	$-[Cys-Gly-His-Cys]_2-$
Ca binding protein 1 (Erp72)	72	ER	$-[Cys-Gly-His-Cys]_3-$
Phospholipase C gamma (PLCγ)	61	ER	$-[Cys-Gly-His-Cys]_2-$
Macrophage migration inhibitory factor (MIF)	12	EX	-Cys-Ala-Leu-Cys-

NOTE: Mt: mitochondria, ER: endoplasmic reticulum, EX: extracellular/intracellular.

in protection against apoptosis in mitochondria.[36] As both TRX and TRX-2 are known regulators of the manifestation of apoptosis under redox-sensitive caspase, their actions may be coordinated. However, the functions of TRX-1 and TRX-2 do not seem to compensate for each other completely, since TRX-2 knockout (KO) mice were found be embryonically lethal.[35]

It is known that many TRX family molecules, such as protein disulfide isomerases (PDIs), are localized in the endoplasmic reticulum. The transmembrane TRX-related protein (TMX) was reported as a novel transmembrane TRX-family molecule localized in the endoplasmic reticulum,[37] and may be related to endoplasmic reticulum stress.[38] Glutaredoxin (GRX) is another example of the TRX family of molecules, which has GSH-disulfide oxidoreductase activity with a TRX-like domain. GRX reduces low molecular weight disulfides and proteins in association with NADPH and GSH reductase. Macrophage migration inhibitory factor (MIF) is a 12kDa protein with a redox-active sequence, and shows a proinflammatory cytokine function. Recent study shows that MIF inhibits the activity of peroxiredoxin, TRX-dependent peroxidase, which may partly explain the proinflammatory function of MIF.[39] The cysteinylated protein of MIF in Cys60 is a glycosylation inhibiting factor (GIF) with inhibitory effects on IgE production.[40]

TRX BINDING PROTEIN-2 / VITAMIN D UPREGULATED PROTEIN 1

TRX binding protein-2 (TBP-2) identified by yeast two-hybrid screening binds to reduced TRX but not to oxidized TRX.[41] TBP-2 was originally identified as a vitamin D upregulated protein 1 (VDUP1) in HL-60 cells treated with 1,25-dihydroxyvitamin D,[42] and is thought to be a negative regulator of TRX.[41] Several cysteine residues were identified, some of which were assumed to bind the active site of TRX.[43] Therefore, overexpression of TBP-2/VDUP1 may block the action of TRX, eventually leading to the inhibition of cellular proliferation. TBP-2/VDUP1 was isolated from a cDNA library enriched with mRNA species that immediately increased upon administration of BrdU, indicating a senescence-associated gene.[44] Enhanced expression of TBP-2/VDUP1 was also reported to be sensitive to paraquat-induced oxidative stress.[45]

On the other hand, a significant reduction in TBP-2/VDUP1 expression was observed in several tumor cell lines and tumor tissues, including human primary breast and colon tumors.[46,47] We reported that expression of TBP-2/VDUP1 was lost in HTLV-I-positive IL-2-dependent cell lines but maintained in HTLV-I-negative T cells. Introducing TBP-2/VDUP1 into HTLV-I-positive T cell lines significantly suppressed cellular proliferation as indicated by the formation of formazan. We also observed that cell cycle arrest occurred at the G_1 stage in association with an increase of p16 expression and reduction of Rb phosphorylation in TBP-2/VDUP1–overexpressing cells.[48] Moreover, a strong anti-oncogenic HDAC inhibitor, suberoylanilide hydroxamic acid (SAHA), upregulated the expression of TBP-2/VDUP1, accompanied by a significant reduction in TRX.[46]

When cells are severely damaged by ROS generation or other biological stresses, cellular proliferation has been shown to be completely blocked at the G_1/G_0 stage. Typical phenotypes of cells under cell cycle arrest virtually simulated multiple aspects of cellular aging or senescence. Indeed, several genetic mutations have been identified to show shorter life spans if continuous cellular proliferation is inhibited by DNA damage,[49] DNA repair defects,[50–52] enhanced apoptosis,[53] or decreased telomere length.[54,55] These reports support the idea that the expression of TRX and TBP-2/VDUP1 are complementarily reflected in cellular proliferation and cellular senescence *in vivo* and *in vitro* (FIG. 2). Recently, spontaneous mutation at the locus *Hyplip1* was reported to be linked to familial combined hyperlipidemia, and the corresponding nonsense mutation was found to be within the coding region of Txnip, which is identical to TBP-2/VDUP1.[56] Indeed, a reduction of Txnip mRNA expression clearly resulted in an increase in the concentration of plasma triglycerides.[56, 57] These studies strongly suggest that the putative biological function of TBP-2/VDUP1 may also be involved in the regulation of lipid metabolism. We are currently investigating the biological roles of

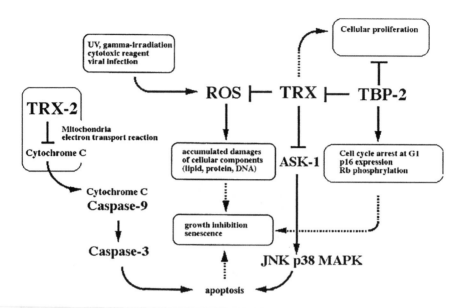

FIGURE 2. Multiple functions of TRX and TBP-2 in oxidative stress during the aging process. TRX, TRX-2, and TBP-2 are involved in a variety of signal transduction pathways, including ROS-mediated cellular damage and apoptosis. The accumulated damage of cellular components eventually leads to inhibition of growth and cellular senescence. Abbreviations: ROS, reactive oxygen species; TRX, thioredoxin; TBP-2, thioredoxin binding protein-2; ASK-1, apoptosis signal-regulating kinase 1; JNK, c-Jun N-terminal kinase.

TBP-2/VDUP1 in the regulation of energy metabolism and life span using TBP-2/VDUP1 genetically modified animals.

CONCLUDING REMARKS

In conclusion, TRX is a strong redox-regulating anti-oxidant protein that has significant quenching capability against induced oxidative stress. TRX-overexpressing transgenic mice showed not only stronger resistance to inflammatory reactions in primary host defense but also cytoprotective effects against oxidative stress by scavenging ROS. Moreover, TRX-overexpressing transgenic mice can achieve significantly extended life span. The expression of TBP-2/VDUP1, a negative regulator of TRX, is frequently associated with suppressed growth conditions of cellular proliferation. The enhanced expression of TBP-2/VDUP1 demonstrated cell cycle arrest at the G_1 stage and possibly mimicked cellular aging with the expression of p16. Taken together,

TRX and TBP-2/VDUP1 can serve as index markers for cellular proliferation and senescence based on their correlative expressions with cellular redox conditions.

ACKNOWLEDGMENTS

We thank Ms. Y. Kanekiyo for secretarial help. This work was partially supported by a grant from a Grant-in-Aid for Scientific Research from the Ministry of Education, Culture, Sports, Science and Technology, Japan, and by the Research and Development Program for New Bio-Industry Initiatives.

REFERENCES

1. HONDA, Y. & S. HONDA. 2002. Oxidative stress and life span determination in the nematode *Caenorhabditis elegans*. Ann. N.Y. Acad Sci. **959:** 466–474.
2. LARSEN, P.L. 1993. Aging and resistance to oxidative damage in *Caenorhabditis elegans*. Proc. Natl. Acad. Sci. USA **90:** 8905–8909.
3. SCOTT, B.A., M.S. AVIDAN & C.M. CROWDER. 2002. Regulation of hypoxic death in *C. elegans* by the insulin/IGF receptor homolog DAF-2. Science **296:** 2388–2391.
4. HONDA, Y. & S. HONDA. 1999. The daf-2 gene network for longevity regulates oxidative stress resistance and Mn-superoxide dismutase gene expression in *Caenorhabditis elegans*. FASEB J. **13:** 1385–1393.
5. FENG, J., F. BUSSIERE & S. HEKIMI. 2001. Mitochondrial electron transport is a key determinant of life span in *Caenorhabditis elegans*. Dev. Cell. **1:** 633–644.
6. ISHII, N. *et al.* 1998. A mutation in succinate dehydrogenase cytochrome b causes oxidative stress and ageing in nematodes. Nature **394:** 694–697.
7. KAYSER, E. B. *et al.* 2001. Mitochondrial expression and function of GAS-1 in *Caenorhabditis elegans*. J. Biol. Chem. **276:** 20551–20558.
8. LAKOWSKI, B. & S. HEKIMI. 1996. Determination of life-span in *Caenorhabditis elegans* by four clock genes. Science **272:** 1010–1013.
9. LIN, Y. J., L. SEROUDE & S. BENZER. 1998. Extended life-span and stress resistance in the *Drosophila* mutant methuselah. Science **282:** 943–946.
10. ORR, W.C. & R.S. SOHAL. 1994. Extension of life-span by overexpression of superoxide dismutase and catalase in *Drosophila melanogaster*. Science **263:** 1128–1130.
11. RUAN, H. *et al.* 2002. High-quality life extension by the enzyme peptide methionine sulfoxide reductase. Proc. Natl. Acad. Sci. USA **99:** 2748–2753.
12. PARKERS, T.L. *et al.* 1998. Extension of *Drosophila* lifespan by overexpression of human SOD1 in motor neurons. Nat. Genet. **19:** 171–174.
13. MIGLIACCIO, E. *et al.* 1999. The p66shc adaptor protein controls oxidative stress response and life span in mammals. Nature **402:** 309–313.
14. NAPOLI, C. *et al.* 2003. Deletion of the p66Shc longevity gene reduces systemic and tissue oxidative stress, vascular cell apoptosis, and early atherogenesis in mice fed a high-fat diet. Proc. Natl. Acad. Sci. USA **100:** 2112–2116.

15. MOSKOVITZ, J. *et al.* 2001. Methionine sulfoxide reductase (MsrA) is a regulator of antioxidant defense and lifespan in mammals. Proc. Natl. Acad. Sci. USA. **98:** 12920–12925.
16. TAGAYA, Y. *et al.* 1989. ATL-derived factor (ADF), an IL-2 receptor/Tac inducer homologous to thioredoxin; possible involvement of dithiol-reduction in the IL-2 receptor induction. EMBO J. **8:** 757–764.
17. OKAMOTO, T. *et al.* 1992. Human thioredoxin/adult T cell leukemia-derived factor activates the enhancer binding protein of human immunodeficiency virus type 1 by thiol redox control mechanism. Int. Immunol. **4:** 811–819.
18. WAKASUGI, H. *et al.* 1987. Epstein-Barr virus-containing B-cell line produces an interleukin 1 that it uses as a growth factor. Proc. Natl. Acad. Sci. USA **84:** 804–808.
19. HOLMGREN, A. 1985. Thioredoxin. Annu. Rev. Biochem. **54:** 237–271.
20. MULLER, E.G. 1991. Thioredoxin deficiency in yeast prolongs S phase and shortens the G1 interval of the cell cycle. J. Biol. Chem. **266:** 9194–9202.
21. SALZ, H.K. *et al.* 1994. The *Drosophila* maternal effect locus deadhead encodes a thioredoxin homolog required for female meiosis and early embryonic development. Genetics **136:** 1075–1086.
22. MATSUI, M. *et al.* 1996. Early embryonic lethality caused by targeted disruption of the mouse thioredoxin gene. Dev. Biol. **178:** 179–185.
23. AKAMATSU, Y. *et al.* 1997. Redox regulation of the DNA binding activity in transcription factor PEBP2. The roles of two conserved cysteine residues. J. Biol. Chem. **272:** 14497–14500.
24. UENO, M. *et al.* 1999. Thioredoxin-dependent redox regulation of p53-mediated p21 activation. J. Biol. Chem. **274:** 35809–35815.
25. SAITOH, M. *et al.* 1998. Mammalian thioredoxin is a direct inhibitor of apoptosis signal-regulating kinase (ASK) 1. EMBO J. **17:** 2596–2606.
26. LESLIE, N.R. *et al.* 2003. Redox regulation of PI 3-kinase signalling via inactivation of PTEN. EMBO J. **22:** 5501–5510.
27. TAKAGI, Y. *et al.* 1999. Overexpression of thioredoxin in transgenic mice attenuates focal ischemic brain damage. Proc. Natl. Acad. Sci. USA **96:** 4131–4136.
28. NAKAMURA, H. *et al.* 2002. Enhhanced resistancy of thioredoxin-transgenic mice against influenza virus-induced pneumonia. Immunol. Lett. **82:** 165–170.
29. HOSHINO, T. *et al.* 2003. Redox-active protein thioredoxin prevents proinflammatory cytokine- or bleomycin-induced lung injury. Am. J. Respir. Crit. Care Med. **168:** 1075–1083.
30. SHIOJI, K. *et al.* 2002. Overexpression of thioredoxin-1 in transgenic mice attenuates adriamycin-induced cardiotoxicity. Circulation **106:** 1403–1409.
31. NAKAMURA, H. *et al.* 2001. Circulating thioredoxin suppresses lipopolysaccharide-induced neutrophil chemotaxis. Proc. Natl. Acad. Sci. USA **98:** 15143–15148.
32. MITSUI, A. *et al.* 2002. Overexpression of human thioredoxin in transgenic mice controls oxidative stress and life span. Antioxid. Redox Signal. **4:** 693–696.
33. SPYROU, G., *et al.* 1997. Cloning and expression of a novel mammalian thioredoxin. J. Biol. Chem. **272:** 2936–2941.
34. TANAKA, T. *et al.* 2002. Thioredoxin-2 (TRX-2) is an essential gene regulating mitochondria-dependent apoptosis. EMBO J. **21:** 1695–1703.
35. NONN, L., *et al.* 2003. The absence of mitochondrial thioredoxin 2 causes massive apoptosis, exencephaly, and early embryonic lethality in homozygous mice. Mol. Cell. Biol. **23:** 916–922.

36. CHEN, Y. *et al.* 2002. Overexpressed human mitochondrial thioredoxin confers resistance to oxidant-induced apoptosis in human osteosarcoma cells. J. Biol. Chem. **277:** 33242–33248.
37. MATSUO, Y. *et al.* 2001. Identification of a novel thioredoxin-related transmembrane protein. J. Biol. Chem. **276:** 10032–10038.
38. MATSUO, Y. *et al.* 2004. TMX, a human transmembrane oxidoreductase of the thioredoxin family: the possible role in disulfide-linked protein folding in the endoplasmic reticulum. Arch. Biochem. Biophys. **423:** 81–87.
39. JUNG, H. *et al.* 2001. Regulation of macrophage migration inhibitory factor and thiol-specific antioxidant protein PAG by direct interaction. J. Biol. Chem. **276:** 15504–15510.
40. WATARAI, H. *et al.* 2000. Posttranslational modification of the glycosylation inhibiting factor (GIF) gene product generates bioactive GIF. Proc. Natl. Acad. Sci. USA **97:** 13251–13256.
41. NISHIYAMA, A. *et al.* 1999. Identification of thioredoxin-binding protein-2/ vitamin D(3) up-regulated protein 1 as a negative regulator of thioredoxin function and expression. J. Biol. Chem. **274:** 21645–21650.
42. CHEN, K. S. & H. F. DELUCA. 1994. Isolation and characterization of a novel cDNA from HL-60 cells treated with 1,25-dihydroxyvitamin D-3. Biochim. Biophys. Acta. **1219:** 26–32.
43. YAMANAKA, H. *et al.* 2000. A possible interaction of thioredoxin with VDUP1 in HeLa cells detected in a yeast two-hybrid system. Biochem. Biophys. Res. Commun. **271:** 796–800.
44. SUZUKI, T. *et al.* 2001. Induction of senescence-associated genes by 5-bromodeoxyuridine in HeLa cells. Exp. Gerontol. **36:** 465–474.
45. JOGUCHI, A. *et al.* 2002. Overexpression of VDUP1 mRNA sensitizes HeLa cells to paraquat. Biochem. Biophys. Res. Commun. **293:** 293–297.
46. BUTLER, L.M. *et al.* 2002. The histone deacetylase inhibitor SAHA arrests cancer cell growth, up-regulates thioredoxin-binding protein-2, and down-regulates thioredoxin. Proc. Natl. Acad. Sci. USA. **99:** 11700–11705.
47. YANG, X., L.H. YOUNG & J.M. VOIGT. 1998. Expression of a vitamin D–regulated gene (VDUP-1) in untreated- and MNU-treated rat mammary tissue. Breast Cancer Res. Treat. **48:** 33–44.
48. NISHINAKA, Y. *et al.* 2004. Loss of thioredoxin-binding protein-2/vitamin D3 up-regulated protein 1 in human T-cell leukemia virus type I-dependent T cell transformation: implications for adult T-cell leukemia leukemogenesis. Cancer Res. **64:** 1287–1292.
49. DOLLE, M.E. *et al.* 1997. Rapid accumulation of genome rearrangements in liver but not in brain of old mice. Nat. Genet. **17:** 431–434.
50. DE BOER, J. *et al.* 2002. Premature aging in mice deficient in DNA repair and transcription. Science **296:** 1276–1279.
51. VOGEL, H. *et al.* 1999. Deletion of Ku86 causes early onset of senescence in mice. Proc. Natl. Acad. Sci. USA **96:** 10770–10775.
52. YU, C.E. *et al.* 1996. Positional cloning of the Werner's syndrome gene. Science **272:** 258–262.
53. TYNER, S.D. *et al.* 2002. p53 mutant mice that display early ageing-associated phenotypes. Nature **415:** 45–53.
54. HERRERA, E. *et al.* 1999. Disease states associated with telomerase deficiency appear earlier in mice with short telomeres. EMBO J. **18:** 2950–2960.

55. WONG, K. K. *et al.* 2003. Telomere dysfunction and Atm deficiency compromises organ homeostasis and accelerates ageing. Nature **421:** 643–648.
56. BODNAR, J.S. *et al.* 2002. Positional cloning of the combined hyperlipidemia gene Hyplip1. Nat. Genet. **30:** 110–116.
57. CASTELLANI, L.W. *et al.* 1998. Mapping a gene for combined hyperlipidaemia in a mutant mouse strain. Nat. Genet. **18:** 374–377.
58. KAEBERLEIN, M., M. MCVEY & L. GUARENTE. 1999. The SIR2/3/4 complex and SIR2 alone promote longevity in Saccharomyces cerevisiae by two different mechanisms. Genes Dev. **13:** 2570–2580.
59. KWAN KY & J.C. WANG. 2001. Mice lacking DNA topoisomerase IIIbeta develop to maturity but show a reduced mean lifespan. Proc. Natl. Acad. Sci. **98:** 5717–5721.
60. LIN, Y.J., L. SEROUDE & S. BENZER. 1998. Extended life-span and stress resistance in the *Drosophila* mutant methuselah. Science **282:** 943–946.
61. ROGINA B. *et al.* 2000. Extended life-span conferred by cotransporter gene mutations in *Drosophila*. Science **290:** 2137–2140.
62. SUN, J. *et al.* 2002. Induced overexpression of mitochondrial Mn-superoxide dismutase extends the life span of adult *Drosophila melanogaster*. Genetics **161:** 661–672.
63. JOHNSON, T.E. 1990. Increased life-span of age-1 mutants in *Caenorhabditis elegans* and lower Gompertz rate of aging. Science **249:** 908–912.
64. KIMURA, K.D., *et al.* 1997. daf-2, an insulin receptor-like gene that regulates longevity and diapause in *Caenorhabditis elegans*. Science **277:** 942–946.
65. LIN, K. *et al.* 1997. daf-16: An HNF-3/forkhead family member that can function to double the life-span of *Caenorhabditis elegans*. Science **278:** 1319–1322.
66. TATAR, M. *et al.* 2001. A mutant *Drosophila* insulin receptor homolog that extends life-span and impairs neuroendocrine function. Science **292:** 107–110.
67. CLANCY, D.J. *et al.* 2001. Extension of life-span by loss of CHICO, a *Drosophila* insulin receptor substrate protein. Science **292:** 104–106.
68. ZHOU, Y. *et al.* 1997. A mammalian model for Laron syndrome produced by targeted disruption of the mouse growth hormone receptor/binding protein gene (the Laron mouse). Proc. Natl. Acad. Sci. USA **94:** 13215–13220.
69. BLUHER, M., B.B. KAHN & C.R. KAHN. 2003 Extended longevity in mice lacking the insulin receptor in adipose tissue. Science **299:** 572–574.
70. HOLZENBERGER, M. *et al.* 2003. IGF-1 receptor regulates lifespan and resistance to oxidative stress in mice. Nature **421:**182–187.

The Different Paths to Age One Hundred

THOMAS PERLS

Geriatrics Section, New England Centenarian Study, Department of Medicine, Boston University Medical Center, Boston, Massacuhetts 02118, USA

ABSTRACT: Attaining age 100 is a rare event in industrialized nations, occurring in 1 person per 10,000 in the population. Becoming a centenarian does not appear to be rare because the individual genetic or behavioral factors (such as specific genetic polymorphisms or lack of specific toxic exposures) that enable such longevity are rare, but rather because having the adequate combination of these factors is rare.

KEYWORDS: longevity; aging; age-associated disease; morbidity and mortality; geriatrics; gender; gerontology; genetics; inheritance; Alzheimer's disease

MY INTRODUCTION TO CENTENARIANS

As a medical student and a physician in training, my experiences with hospitalized older patients and the conventional wisdom of the time reinforced for me the notion that the older you get, the sicker you get. When I came across two centenarians in the course of my clinical work as a geriatrics fellow, I had the preconceived notion that centenarians would have every age-related disease under the sun, particularly Alzheimer's disease, and that given their age, they would be at death's doorstep. To my surprise, and very lucky for me, the two centenarians in my practice were in very good shape. Soon thereafter, we began the New England Centenarian Study (NECS), a population-based study of all the centenarians in eight towns around Boston with the following hypothesis: Centenarians achieve their age by virtue of aging slowly and markedly delaying or escaping the diseases associated with aging.[1,2] There are numerous definitions of what "aging slowly" might mean. One definition that I like is: a decreased rate of decline in adaptive capacity or functional reserve, and therefore a decreased vulnerability. It would seem to make

Address for correspondence: Thomas Perls, M.D., M.P.H., Geriatrics Section, New England Centenarian Study, Department of Medicine, Boston University Medical Center, Robinson 2400, 88 East Newton Street, Boston, MA 02118. Voice 617-638-6688; fax: 617-638-6671.
thperls@bu.edu

Ann. N.Y. Acad. Sci. 1055: 13–25 (2005). © 2005 New York Academy of Sciences.
doi: 10.1196/annals.1323.004

sense that persons who developed a stroke, heart attack, or Alzheimer's disease in their 60s or 70s would be unlikely to be able to go on the extra 30 or 40 years to age 100.

COMPRESSION OF DISABILITY

We have since found that a substantial proportion of centenarians do not delay age-related illnesses, but they appear to postpone disability to very advanced ages. In the New England Centenarian Study, we observed that 90% of centenarians were independently functioning at the mean age of 92 years.[3] Most subjects experienced a decline in their cognitive function only in the last 3 to 5 years of their lives.[4,5] Further examination of the ages of onset for ten common age-associated diseases (hypertension, heart disease, diabetes, stroke, non–skin and skin cancer, osteoporosis, thyroid condition, Parkinson's disease, chronic obstructive pulmonary disease, and cataracts) among 424 centenarians (323 males and 101 females) revealed that the centenarians fit into three morbidity profiles: "survivors," "delayers," and "escapers."[6] Survivors, individuals who were diagnosed with age-related illness prior to age 80, accounted for 24% of the male and 43% of the female centenarians ($P = 0.0009$). Delayers, individuals in whom the onset of age-related diseases was delayed until at least age 80, accounted for 44% of the male and 42% of female centenarians. Escapers, individuals who attained the 100th year of life without the diagnosis of an age-related disease, accounted for 32% of the male and 15% of the female centenarians ($P = 0.0003$). The finding of a substantial number of centenarians fitting a "survivor" profile may be inconsistent with the compression-of-morbidity hypothesis. That most centenarians appear to be functionally independent through their early 90s suggests the possibility that "survivors" and "delayers" are better able to cope with illnesses and remain functionally independent. Thus, in the case of centenarians, it may be more accurate to note a compression of disability rather than of morbidity. This is not the case, as would be expected with illnesses associated with high mortality risk. When examining only the most lethal diseases of the elderly, including heart disease, non–skin cancer, and stroke, 87% of males and 83% of females delayed or escaped these diseases.

Typically 85% of centenarians are female and 15% are male. As noted above, however, even though male centenarians are fewer in number, they tend to be functionally more fit than their female counterparts. The reason for this apparent paradox may be that, for unclear reasons, women are physiologically stronger than men when it comes to maladies associated with aging. Women thus carry a double-edged sword of living longer with diseases associated with aging rather than dying from them relative to men. We hypothesize that men, on the other hand, must be relatively disease-free in order to reach 100. Generally speaking, the male centenarians in our study are functionally doing well, and when they do develop a significant health problem, their mortality risk rises quickly, particularly relative to similarly aged women.

These results suggest there may be multiple routes to achieving exceptional longevity and that there are gender differences according to which route is taken. These routes represent different phenotypes and thus likely different genotypes of centenarians. The identification of three subtypes of centenarians, *survivors, delayers*, and *escapers*, provides direction for future study into factors that determine exceptional longevity.[6]

PATHOLOGICALLY DEFINING "DISEASE-FREE" AGING

Among subjects noted to fit the escaper category, a number of centenarian subjects have provided the study with the tremendous gift of donating their brains for postmortem study. Our first subject to do so illustrated the concept of pathologically disease-free aging. This woman, at age 100 years, performed within the norms of a 60-year-old on the NECS battery of neuropsychological examinations.[4] Approximately nine months after testing she died owing to a cardiac event. We considered two possibilities of what to expect from her brain autopsy results: (1) that she would have many of the neuritic plaques and neurofibrillary tangles associated with Alzheimer's disease, but somehow had some nondescript adaptive capacity or functional reserve that would allow her to not manifest the disease clinically and (2) that her brain would not reveal any of these neuropathological markers that numerous scientists felt were a normal consequence of extreme old age. In fact, pathological examination of the brain demonstrated the absence of neurofibrillary tangles or neuritic plaques. Since this autopsy, the NECS has had four other subjects like this, where there was a very good correlation between the subject's normal clinical presentation and his or her lack of neuropathology. Of course, there are other people who have a substantial amount of neurofibrillary tangles and neuritic plaques but do not clinically manifest cognitive impairment. At least in the case of subjects revealing no neuropathological markers of disease, these individuals appear to be examples of disease-free aging. There is obviously quite a spectrum. Had the above subject had the opportunity to live to 119 years, for example (like our oldest-ever subject who underwent autopsy), she might have then demonstrated vascular disease and signs of AD, both clinically and pathologically.

EXTREMES OF THE EXTREME

Approximately one per 10,000 Americans is a centenarian. Within this group are even more rare individuals, super-centenarians, who are people ages 110 years and older. There are probably about 250 super-centenarians in the United States, or one per ten million. Another interesting group, the rarest of the rare, are centenarians who have had everything equivalent to an atomic bomb thrown at their bodies and they are still getting to age 100 in good health. We have a handful of subjects in the NECS who have smoked three packs a day for 50 years without clinical evidence of heart disease, stroke, Alzheimer's disease or cancer. Humorously, one of these subjects remarked that it was the three martinis a day he was drinking that "did the trick." If one wants to look for protective genetic factors, their best chances may be investigating these individuals who must have had some protective factors in order to counteract such exposures that otherwise carry such a high mortality rate. Perhaps, 20 or 30 years ago, 100-year-olds might have represented enough of an extreme, but now, given recent medical and other interventions, such inherent protective factors might not be necessary for survival to 100, but are possibly still necessary for survival to 110.

FACTORS ASSOCIATED WITH EXCEPTIONAL LONGEVITY

The relative contribution of environmental and genetic influences to longevity has been a source of debate. Assessing heritability in 10,505 Swedish twin pairs reared together and apart, Ljungquist and colleagues attributed 35% of the variance in longevity to genetic influences and 65% of the variance to non-shared environmental effects.[7] Other twin studies indicate heritability estimates of life expectancy between 25% and 30%.[8,9] A study of 1,655 Old Order Amish subjects born between 1749 and 1890 and surviving beyond age 30 years resulted in a heritability calculation of 0.25 for life span.[10] These studies support the contention that the life spans of average humans with their average set of genetic polymorphisms are differentiated primarily by their habits and environments. Supporting this idea is a study of Seventh Day Adventists. In contrast to the American average life expectancy of 78 years, the average life expectancy of Seventh Day Adventists is 88 years. Because of their religious beliefs, members of this religious faith maintain optimal health habits such as not smoking, a vegetarian diet, regular exercise, and maintenance of a lean body mass that translate into the addition of 10 years to their average life expectancy compared to that of other Americans.[11] Given that in the United States, 75% of Americans are overweight and one-third of those are obese,[12] far too many people still use tobacco,[13] and far too few persons regularly exercise,[14] it is no wonder that the American average life expectancy is about 10 years less than what our average set of genetic variations should be able to achieve for us.

Of course there are exceptions to the rule. There are individuals who have genetic profiles with or without prerequisite environmental exposures that predispose them to diseases at younger ages. There is also the component of luck, which, good or bad, plays a role in life expectancy. And finally, there is the possibility that genetic and environmental factors exist that facilitate the ability to live to ages significantly older than what the average set of genetic and environmental exposures normally allows. Because the oldest individuals in the twin studies were in their early to mid-80s, those studies provide information about heritability of average life expectancy, but not for those of substantially older ages (e.g., 100 years and older). As discussed below, to survive the 15 or more years beyond what our average set of genetic variations is capable of achieving for us, it appears that people need to have benefited from a relatively rare combination of what might be not so rare environmental, behavioral, and genetic characteristics and that a number of these factors appear to be shared within families.

THE FAMILIALITY OF EXCEPTIONAL LONGEVITY

Studying Mormon pedigrees from the Utah Population Database, Kerber and colleagues investigated the impact of family history upon the longevity of 78,994 individuals who achieved at least the age of 65 years.[15] The relative risk of survival (λ_s) calculated for siblings of probands achieving the 97th percentile of "excess longevity" (for males this corresponded to an age of 95 years, and for women to an age of 97 years) was 2.30. Recurrence risks among more distant relatives in the Mormon pedigrees remained significantly greater than 1.0 for numerous classes of relatives, leading to the conclusion that single-gene effects were at play in this survival advantage. The Mormon study findings closely agree with a study of the Icelandic population in which first-degree relatives of those living to the 95th percentile of surviving age were almost twice as likely to also live to the 95th percentile of survival compared with controls.[16] Both research groups asserted that the range of recurrent relative risks that they observed indicated a substantial genetic component to exceptional longevity.

To further explore the genetic aspects of exceptional old age, we studied 444 centenarian pedigrees containing 2,092 siblings.[17] We compared sibling death rates and survival probabilities with national U.S. death rates and survival probabilities according to the Social Security Administration's life table for the cohort born in 1900. Compared with the 1900 birth cohort, the siblings of centenarians maintained a life-long reduction in risk for death of approximately one-half, even up through very old age.

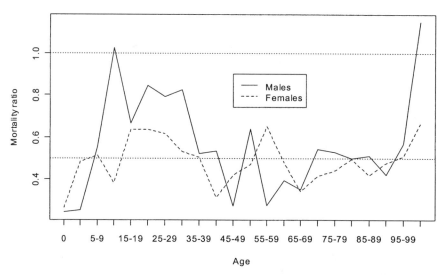

FIGURE 1. Relative mortality of male and female siblings of centenarians compared with birth cohort–matched individuals (controls) from the general American population. (Survival experience of the controls comes from the Social Security Administration's 1900 birth-cohort life table.)

As shown in FIGURE 1, female siblings had death rates at all ages that were about one-half the average for their birth cohort; male siblings had a similar advantage at most ages, though diminished somewhat during adolescence and young adulthood. The siblings had an average age of death of 76.7 for females and 70.4 for males compared to 58.3 and 51.5 for the general population. Even after accounting for race and education, the net survival advantage of siblings of centenarians was found to be 16 years greater than that of the general population. Siblings may share environmental and behavioral factors early in life that have strong effects throughout life. It would make sense that some of these effects are primarily responsible for the shared survival advantage up to middle age. Alternatively, some of these effects might not become evident until after middle age.

Recent evidence of effects of early life conditions on adult morbidity and mortality points to the importance of adopting a life course perspective in studies of chronic morbidity and mortality in later life as well as in investigations of exceptional longevity.[18–25] Characteristics of childhood environment are not only associated with morbidity and mortality at middle age, but they have also been found to predict survival to extreme old age.[26,27] Stone analyzed effects of childhood conditions on survival to extreme old age among cohorts born during the late 19th century.[28] Key factors predicting survival from childhood to age 110+ for these individuals, most of whom were born between 1870 and 1889, were farm residence, presence of both parents in the household, American-born parents, family ownership of its dwelling, residence in a rural area and residence in the non-South—characteristics similar to those that had been previously shown to predict survival to age 85.[26,27]

In general however, environmental characteristics, such as socioeconomic status, lifestyle, and region of residence, are likely to diverge as siblings grow older. Thus, if the survival advantage of the siblings of centenarians is mainly due to environmental factors, that advantage should decline with age. In contrast, the stability of relative risk for death across a wide age range suggests that the advantage is due more to genetic than to environmental factors.

Whereas death rates reflect the current intensity of death at a moment in time, survival probability reflects the cumulative experience of death up to that moment in a cohort's life history. Thus, a relatively constant advantage from moment to moment (as seen in the relative death rates) translates into an increasing survival advantage over a lifetime (as seen in the relative survival probabilities). This is seen in TABLE 1, which shows the relative survival probabilities of the male and female siblings of centenarians at various ages.

By the age of 100 years, the relative survival probability for siblings of centenarians is 8.2 for women and 17 for men. From the analysis of death rates, we know that the siblings' survival advantage does not increase as the siblings age. Rather, the siblings' relative probability of survival is a cumulative measure and reflects their life-long survival advantage over the general population born around the same time. The marked increase in relative survival probability and sustained survival advantage in extreme old age could be consistent with the forces of demographic selection, in which genes or environmental factors (or both) that predispose to longevity win out over those that are associated with premature or average mortality. The substantially higher relative survival probability values for men at older ages might reflect the fact that male mortality rates are substantially higher than female mortality rates at these ages and, thus, that men gain a greater advantage from beneficial genotypes than women do. Another possibility is that men require an even more rare combination of genetic and environmental factors to achieve extreme age than women do.[29] Either possibility could explain why men make up only 15% of centenarians.

So is the ability to reach 100 years of age a matter of some fountain-of-aging-well gene or other rare factor (which would thus explain why centenarians are also so rare)? More than likely not, and I must say that a significant portion of my thinking about this has been influenced by Dr. George Martin of the University of Washington in Seattle.[30] It is difficult to imagine genetic factors that would impart twice the survival advantage among people in their 20s or 30s compared to their birth-cohort peers. Certainly such individuals would not be predisposed to very rare childhood genetic diseases, but those only involve a small minority of the population. Rather, such a survival advantage at young ages would be due to avoiding the 1919 influenza epidemic,

TABLE 1. RSP with 95% confidence intervals (CI) of siblings of centenarians versus U.S. 1900 cohort

	Males			Females		
	RSP	Lower 95% CI	Upper 95% CI	RSP	Lower 95% CI	Upper 95% CI
20	1.00	1.00	1.00	1.00	1.00	1.00
25	1.00	0.99	1.01	1.01	1.00	1.02
60	1.18	1.15	1.21	1.12	1.09	1.14
65	1.29	1.25	1.33	1.16	1.13	1.19
70	1.48	1.42	1.53	1.24	1.21	1.28
75	1.68	1.60	1.77	1.36	1.31	1.41
80	2.03	1.90	2.16	1.54	1.47	1.60
85	2.69	2.47	2.91	1.83	1.73	1.93
90	4.08	3.62	4.54	2.56	2.39	2.74
95	8.35	6.98	9.71	4.15	3.73	4.57
100	17.0	10.8	23.1	8.22	6.55	9.90

better socioeconomic status, avoiding significant obesity, not smoking, and other environmental factors. As one ages into the 40s or 50s, then perhaps it is necessary to have lower risk (environmental and genetic) for heart disease, stroke, hypertension, cancer, and so on. By the time one is in the 80s or 90s, then perhaps, much more controversially, it may be important to have genetic variations that impart some kind of protective effect over the course of one's life that would allow a person who otherwise had the average set of variations facilitating his or her ability to survive to the mid- to late 80s, to then go on to achieve the extra 15 or so years to age 100. Thus perhaps centenarians are so rare at 1 person per 10,000 people because they won the lottery; that is, they had the right combination of all these factors at the right time in their lives.

DECIPHERING GENETIC FACTORS RELATED TO EXCEPTIONAL LONGEVITY

It is practically intuitive to state that centenarians outlive those who are relatively predisposed to age-related fatal illnesses and that they are less likely to have environmental and genetic exposures that contribute to death at earlier ages. This selection phenomenon, called demographic selection, is exemplified by the fact that the apolipoprotein E ε4 allele, associated with heart disease and Alzheimer's disease, is rare in centenarians, whereas the prevalence of an alternative allele, ε2, is relatively high.[31] Along the same lines, it is likely that there are certain environmental exposures that are rare among centenarians as well, such as tobacco, obesity, and bullets. Richard Cutler, in what is now a classic paper in gerontology, proposed that persons who achieve extreme old age do so in great part because they have genetic variations that affect the basic mechanisms of aging and that result in a uniform decreased susceptibility to age-associated diseases.[32] Our studies and those of others researching the oldest old have noted that persons who achieve extreme old age probably lack many of the variations (the "disease genes") that substantially increase risk for premature death by predisposing persons to various fatal diseases, both age-associated and non–age-associated.[33] More controversial is the idea that genetic variations might confer protection against the basic mechanisms of aging or age-related illnesses (the "longevity-enabling genes").[34] The progressive selecting out of more and more genetically fit persons of very old age lays the foundation for a simpler model for sorting out the genetics of aging and longevity.

The discovery of genetic variations that explain even 5% to 10% of the variation in survival to extreme old age could yield important clues about the cellular and biochemical mechanisms that affect basic mechanisms of aging and susceptibility to age-associated diseases. The elevated relative survival probability values found among the siblings of centenarians (TABLE 1) supported the utility of performing genetic studies to determine what genetic region or regions, and ultimately what genetic variations, centenarians and their siblings have in common that confers their survival advantage.[35] Centenarian sibships from the New England Centenarian Study were included in a genome-wide sibling-pair study of 308 persons belonging to 137 families with exceptional longevity. According to nonparametric analysis, significant evidence for linkage was noted for a locus on chromosome 4, near microsatellite D4S1564.[36]

This interval spanned 12 million base pairs and contained approximately 50 putative genes. In order to identify the specific gene and gene variants having an impact on life span, our genetics colleagues Drs. Annibale Puca, Bard Geesaman, Louis Kunkel, and Mark Daly performed a haplotype-based fine-mapping study of the interval. A detailed haplotype map was created of the chromosome 4 locus that extended over 12 million base pairs and involved the genotyping of more than 2,000 single nucleotide polymorphism (SNP) markers in 700 centenarians and 700 controls. The study identified a haplotype, approximating the gene microsomal transfer protein (MTP), defined by two SNPs that accounted for all of the statistical distortion detected in the region. Statistically, the result appears to be robust, with a relative risk of nearly 2 ($P < 2 \times 10^{-9}$). With interest narrowing in on a single gene, all known SNP polymorphisms for MTP and its promoter were genotyped in 200 centenarians and 200 controls (young individuals). After haplotype reconstruction of the area was completed, a single haplotype, which was underrepresented in the long-lived individuals, accounted for the majority of the statistical distortion at the locus (~15% among the long-lived individuals versus 23% in the controls). MTP plays a first step role in lipoprotein synthesis, combining with APO-B and chylomicrons to form very-low-density lipoprotein (VLDL). This study supports the feasibility of fine-mapping linkage peaks using association studies and the power of using the centenarian genome to identify genes having an impact on longevity and the diseases of aging.[36] In that same study, however, the findings were not replicated in a French referent sample of centenarians, thus raising the possibility that the MTP finding was specific to the collected sample or that it was a false positive finding. Recently Nebel and colleagues[37] conducted an association study to determine whether there were significant differences between nonagenarian and centenarian subjects and controls for the specific MTP variations studied above, and they found no difference. This study again raises the signficant risk of false positive results in association studies and the importance of replicating findings in other sample comparisons. This does not mean that the MTP findings should be altogether discarded. In the Geesamen study, other factors may have been present and common among the experimental group that were linked to the MTP variation or that occurred in combination with it that were responsible for the positive association. Thus there may be an important longevity-associated factor related to MTP that has yet to be uncovered.

Dr. Nir Barzilai and his colleagues, studying Ashkenazi Jewish centenarians and their families, recently found another cardiovascular pathway and gene that is differentiated between centenarians and controls.[38] In Dr. Barzilai's study, controls are the spouses of the centenarians' children. They noted that high-density lipoprotein (HDL) and low-density lipoprotein (LDL) particle sizes were significantly larger among the centenarians and their offspring, and the particle size also differentiated between subjects with and without cardiovascular disease, hypertension, and metabolic syndrome. In a candidate gene approach the researchers then searched the literature for genes that have an impact upon HDL and LDL particle size and they came up with hepatic lipase and cholesteryl ester transfer protein (CETP). Comparing centenarians and their offspring against controls, one variation of CETP was noted to be significantly increased among those with or predisposed for exceptional longevity. Given our findings that cardiovascular disease is significantly delayed among the offspring of centenarians and that 88% of centenarians either delay or escape cardiovascular disease and stroke beyond the age of 80 years, it makes sense that the frequency of genetic polymorphisms that play a role in the risk for such diseases (such as apolipoprotein ε-4) would be differentiated between long-lived individuals and the general population.[31,39–42] It should not be surprising that the genetic associations discovered thus far relate to vascular disease. Clearly, because vascular disease is the number one killer of older people, one would expect to see genetic variations and other risk factors related to vascular disease play prominent roles in survival to extreme old age.

WHAT CAN WE DO RIGHT NOW?

The twin studies and the Adventist Health Study indicate that given the average set of genetic and environmental variations, the majority of people should be able to survive to their mid-80s. Similar to what centenarians experience, it is likely that, were people able to achieve an average life expectancy of approximately 85 years, they would necessarily compress the time during which they experience functional decline towards the end of their lives. Again, the Seventh Day Adventist lifestyle entails being lean, exercising, a vegetarian diet, and not smoking or drinking alcohol (though some studies support drinking a little alcohol).

In the meantime, careful phenotyping of numerous animal and human models of aging, the collection of genetic material, and the current explosion in molecular genetics data and techniques are likely to soon fill important gaps in the aging puzzle. Complex gene–gene and gene–environment interactions will certainly complicate our ability to understand how genes affect aging. However, with the power of demographic selection, centenarians have already proven helpful in deciphering some polymorphisms and genetic loci associated or not associated with exceptional old age. The children of centenarians, who seem to be following closely in their parents' footsteps, might yield additional discoveries about phenotypic and genetic correlates of successful aging.

REFERENCES

1. PERLS, T.T., K. BOCHEN, M. FREEMAN, *et al.* 1999. Validity of reported age and centenarian prevalence in New England. Age Ageing **28:** 193–197.
2. PERLS, T. 1995. The oldest old. Sci. Amer. **272:** 70–75.
3. HITT, R., Y. YOUNG-XU, M. SILVER & T. PERLS. 1999. Centenarians: the older you get, the healthier you have been. Lancet **354:** 652.
4. SILVER, M., K. NEWELL, B. HYMAN, *et al.* 1998. Unraveling the mystery of cognitive changes in old age: correlation of neuropsychological evaluation with neuropathological findings in the extreme old. Int. Psychogeriatr. **10:** 25–41.
5. PERLS, T. 1997. Symposium: Cognitive and functional status of centenarians: reports from four studies. Gerontologist **37:** 37.
6. EVERT, J., E. LAWLER, H. BOGAN & T. PERLS. 2003. Morbidity profiles of centenarians: survivors, delayers, and escapers. J. Gerontol. A Biol. Sci. Med. Sci. **58:** 232–237.
7. LJUNGQUIST, B., S. BERG, J. LANKE, *et al.* 1998. The effect of genetic factors for longevity: a comparison of identical and fraternal twins in the Swedish Twin Registry. J. Gerontol. A Biol. Sci. Med. Sci. **53:** M441–446.
8. HERSKIND, A.M., M. MCGUE, N.V. HOLM, *et al.* 1996. The heritability of human longevity: a population-based study of 2872 Danish twin pairs born 1870-1900. Hum. Genet. **97:** 319–323.

9. McGue, M., J.W. Vaupel, N. Holm & B. Harvald. 1993. Longevity is moderately heritable in a sample of Danish twins born 1870-1880. J. Gerontol. **48:** B237–244.

10. Mitchell, B.D., W.C. Hsueh, T.M. King, *et al.* 2001. Heritability of life span in the Old Order Amish. Am. J. Med. Genet. **102:** 346–352.

11. Fraser, G.E. & D.J. Shavlik. 2001. Ten years of life: is it a matter of choice? Arch. Intern. Med. **161:** 1645–1652.

12. Fontaine, K.R., C. Wang, A.O. Wesfal & D.B. Allison. 2003. Years of life lost to obesity. JAMA **289:** 187–193.

13. Wechsler, H., N.A. Rigotti, J. Gledhill-Hoyt & H. Lee. 1998. Increased levels of cigarette use among college students: a cause for national concern. JAMA **280:** 1673–1678.

14. Wei, M., J.B. Kampert, C.E. Barlow, *et al.* 1999. Relationship between low cardiorespiratory fitness and mortality in normal-weight, overweight, and obese men. JAMA **282:** 1547–1553.

15. Kerber, R.A., E. O'Brien, K.R. Smith & R.M. Cawthon. 2001. Familial excess longevity in Utah genealogies. J. Gerontol. A Biol. Sci. Med. Sci. **56:** B130–139.

16. Gudmundsson, H., D.F. Gudbjartsson, M. Frigge. *et al.* 2000. Inheritance of human longevity in Iceland. Eur. J. Hum. Genet. **8:** 743–749.

17. Perls, T.T., J. Wilmoth, R. Levenson, *et al.* 2002. Life-long sustained mortality advantage of siblings of centenarians. Proc. Natl. Acad. Sci. USA **99:** 8442–8447.

18. Blackwell, D., M.D. Hayward & E.M. Crimmins. 2001. Does childhood health affect chronic morbidity in later life? Soc. Sci. & Med. **52:** 1269–1284.

19. Mosley, W. & R. Gray. 1993. Childhood precursors of adult morbidity and mortality in developing countries: implications for health programs. *In* The Epidemiological Transition: Policy and Planning Implications for Developing Countries. J. Gribble & S. Preston, Eds.: 69–100. National Academy Press. Washington, DC.

20. Elo, I. 1998. Childhood conditions and adult health: evidence from the health and retirement study. Population Aging Research Center Working Papers. University of Pennsylvania Population Aging Research Center. Philadelphia, PA.

21. Barker, D.M. 1998. Babies, Mothers, and Health in Later Life. Churchill Livingstone. London.

22. Kuh, D. & B. Ben-Shlomo. 1997. A Life Course Approach to Chronic Disease Epidemiology. Oxford University Press. Oxford, UK.

23. Costa, D. 2000. Understanding the twentieth century decline in chronic conditions among older men. Demography **37:** 53–72.

24. Hall, A. & C.S. Peekham. 1997. Infections in childhood and pregnancy as a cause of adult disease: methods and examples. Br. Med. Bull. **53:** 10–23.

25. Elford, J., P. Whincup & A.G. Shaper. 1991. Early life experience and adult cardiovascular disease: longitudinal and case-control studies. Int. J. Epidemiol. **20:** 833–844.

26. Preston, S., M.E. Hill & G.L. Drevenstedt. 1998. Childhood conditions that predict survival to advanced ages among African Americans. Soc. Sci. & Med. **47:** 1231–1246.

27. Preston, S., I.T. Elo, M.E. Hill & I. Rosenwaike. 2003. The Demography of African Americans, 1930–1990. Kluwer Academic. Boston.

28. STONE, L. 2002. Early life conditions that predict survival to extreme old age [abstract]. Presented at the Annual Meeting of the Population Association of America, Atlanta, GA.

29. PERLS, T.T. & R. FRETTS. 1998. Why women live longer than men. Scientific American Presents. 9: 100–103.

30. MARTIN, G. 2002. Keynote: mechanisms of senescence—complificationists versus simplificationists. Mech. Ageing Dev. 123: 65–73.

31. SCHACHTER, F., L. FAURE-DELANEF, F. GUENOT, et al. 1994. Genetic associations with human longevity at the APOE and ACE loci. Nat. Genet. 6: 29–32.

32. CUTLER, R.G. 1975. Evolution of human longevity and the genetic complexity governing aging rate. Proc. Natl. Acad. Sci. USA 72: 4664–4668.

33. SCHACHTER, F. 1998. Causes, effects, and constraints in the genetics of human longevity. Am. J. Hum. Genet. 62: 1008–1014.

34. PERLS, T., L.M. KUNKEL & A.A. PUCA. 2002. The genetics of exceptional longevity. J. Am. Geriatr. Soc. 50: 359–368.

35. MCCARTHY, M.I., L. KRUGLYAK & E.S. LANDER. 1998. Sib-pair collection strategies for complex diseases. Genet. Epidemiol. 15: 317–340.

36. PUCA, A.A., M.J. DALY, S.J. BREWSTER, et al. 2001. A genome-wide scan for linkage to human exceptional longevity identifies a locus on chromosome 4. Proc. Natl. Acad. Sci. USA 98: 10505–10508.

37. NEBEL, A., P.J. CROUCHER, R. STIEGLER, et al. 2005. No association between microsomal triglyceride transfer protein (MTP) haplotype and longevity in humans. Proc. Natl. Acad. Sci. USA 102: 7906–7909.

38. BARZILAI, N.A.G., C. SCHECHTER, E.J. SCHAEFER, et al. 2003. Unique lipoprotein phenotype and genotype in humans with exceptional longevity. JAMA 290: 2030–2040.

39. REBECK, G.W., T.T. PERLS, H.L. WEST, et al. 1994. Reduced apolipoprotein epsilon 4 allele frequency in the oldest old Alzheimer's patients and cognitively normal individuals. Neurology 44: 1513–1516.

40. VAN BOCKXMEER, F.M. 1994. ApoE and ACE genes: impact on human longevity. Nat. Genet. 6: 4–5.

41. TILVIS, R.S., T.E. STRANDBERG & K. JUVA. 1998. Apolipoprotein E phenotypes, dementia and mortality in a prospective population sample. J. Am. Geriatr. Soc. 46: 712–715.

42. SMITH, J.D. 2000. Apolipoprotein E4: an allele associated with many diseases. Ann. Med. 32: 118–127.

Genetic Engineering of Mice to Test the Oxidative Damage Theory of Aging

GEORGE M. MARTIN

Department of Pathology, University of Washington, Seattle, Washington 98195, USA

ABSTRACT: The laboratory mouse *Mus musculus domesticus* provides the best current mammalian models for the genetic analysis of aging. We give a brief overview of the use of transgenic manipulations to test the oxidative damage theory of aging. These manipulations are of two types: The first approach engineers mice that exhibit increased *sensitivities* to oxidative damage and thus produces mice that are likely to be short-lived. The second approach engineers mice to be more *resistant* to such injuries, and thus may produce mice that exhibit enhanced longevities, something that is much harder to engineer. The latter result is thus more meaningful, with the caveat that it may result from some special vulnerability of a particular lab strain or lab strains in general. The first approach, most elegantly carried out by Arlan Richardson's laboratory, provides evidence *against* the oxidative damage theory. My colleagues and I have been engaged in the second approach and have accumulated evidence *supporting* the theory. These conventional transgenic experiments, however, should be supplemented by alternative genetic approaches. One that is surprisingly neglected takes advantage of the pleuripotency of embryonic stem cells and the power of somatic cell genetics. A cautionary note is that interventions that minimize oxidative stress may be complicated by unwanted compromises of physiologically adaptive actions such as superoxide signaling and the possible protective effects of certain oxidatively modified proteins.

KEYWORDS: transgenic mice; oxidative damage; somatic cell genetics; catalase; superoxide dismutase; mitochondria

INTRODUCTION

The discovery of constitutional (heritable) genetic variations that modulate the duration of life and various biological markers and disorders of aging have the potential to elucidate the most fundamental aspects of the biology

Address for correspondence: Dr. George M. Martin, Department of Pathology, University of Washington, Seattle, Washington 98195. Voice: 206-543-5088; fax: 206-685-8356.
gmmartin@u.washington.edu

Ann. N.Y. Acad. Sci. 1055: 26–34 (2005). © 2005 New York Academy of Sciences.
doi: 10.1196/annals.1323.005

and pathobiology of aging since, by definition, one is dealing with first principles and not with some downstream epiphenomena. Genetic analysis of tractable model organisms such as *C. elegans* and *D. melanogaster* have been responsible for the elucidation of what appears to be the first biochemical pathway that can be characterized as a "public" mechanism of aging.[1] These investigations have inspired and will continue to inspire mammalian experimental geneticists with major interests in biogerontology, the vast majority of whom work with the common laboratory mouse, *Mus musculus domesticus*.

Our task in this brief review is to summarize the extent to which experiments with transgenic mice have so far contributed support for or against what is arguably the currently most popular fundamental mechanism of aging —the "oxidative damage" or "oxidative stress" or "free radical" theory of aging, as first conceived by Denham Harmon almost a half century ago.[2] We shall confine ourselves to studies that have investigated the "gold standard" for aging studies, namely life-span studies. We conclude that the current evidence is mixed. We also conclude that a particularly promising novel avenue of genetic research, involving somatic cell genetic experiments with cultures of pluripotent mouse embryonic stem cells, is deserving of more attention.

THE OXIDATIVE DAMAGE THEORY OF AGING

Most authors have emphasized mitochondrial electron transport as the essential locus for the generation of reactive oxygen species of importance to the pathobiology of aging. Nature has evolved an elaborate and largely effective system for the quadrivalent reduction of oxygen in the generation of ATP. Fridovich has recently pointed out that previous estimates of the efficiency of that system (~2% "leakiness" via univalent reductions leading to the generation of superoxide anions) were exaggerated because the methodology employed cyanide to block cytochrome *c* oxidase.[3] Nevertheless, a more likely figure of 0.1% univalent reduction may still be insufficient to overcome scavenging enzymes such as superoxide dismutases, glutathione peroxidases, and catalases.[3] One can make a very large list of genetic loci that have the potential to modulate the rates of generation of reactive oxygen species, their scavenging (both enzymatic and nonenzymatic), the relative susceptibilities to damage of the various target organelles and macromolecular assemblies and the degree of their redundancies, the rates of response and the efficiencies of DNA and protein repair mechanisms, the efficiency of the cell cycle regulatory controls to permit healing of DNA damage or, failing such healing, adaptive modes of apoptosis and, finally, the rates and efficiencies of replacement of effete cells via different categories of stem cells and progenitor cells. There is thus a vast repertoire of loci that are potentially rate limiting, in particular genetic backgrounds existing in particular environments, making tests of the theory particularly difficult. Another problem is that not all reactive oxygen species are necessarily pathogenic. Superoxide, for example, can be important in signal transduction processes that play important roles during development. A particularly interesting example has been demonstrated in *Dictiostelium*, in which overexpression of superoxide dismutase inhibits cell aggregation.[4] Moreover, some oxidized proteins may be good for our arteries! In a murine model of atherosclerosis, tyrosyl radical–oxidized high density lipoprotein was found to be more efficient than native high density lipoprotein in the removal of cholesterol from the aorta.[5]

TRANSGENIC MICE THAT ARE MORE SENSITIVE TO OXIDATIVE DAMAGE

The best work to date is that of Holly Van Remmen and colleagues in the Arlan Richardson lab.[6] They used mice heterozygous for a *SOD2* knockout from a line developed by Charles Epstein's lab in a CE1 background (*Sod3*[tm1]*Cje*).[7] These were backcrossed to C57BL/6Jax mice. A special merit of their study was the excellent survival of their wild-type controls, indicative of very good conditions of husbandry. Another attractive feature of the study was the documentation of elevated levels of 8-oxy-2-deoxyguanosine adducts in both nuclear and mitochondrial DNA of both young and old heterozygous SOD2-deficient animals, with the expected comparatively higher levels in mitochondrial DNA for both control and transgenic mice. Also as expected, there was evidence that the SOD2-deficient mice were hypersensitive to paraquat, a generator of superoxide anions. It thus appeared that there would be support for the oxidative damage theory of aging. Yet there was absolutely no evidence of an impact upon the life spans of these SOD2-deficient animals. Moreover, they found no impact of the enzyme deficiency or increased DNA damage upon a few selected biomarkers of aging, including ocular cataracts, the proliferative responses of T and B lymphocytes, and levels of glycoxidation products in skin collagen. One would have to conclude that their experiments provide evidence against the oxidative theory of aging. A peculiar feature of their findings, however, remains unexplained. There was an increased prevalence, in the SOD2-deficient animals, of the same spectrum of neoplasms found in wild-type mice, including the characteristically common lymphomas. Moreover, some 67% of enzyme-deficient animals had multiple tumors, whereas only 18% of controls had such multiple lesions. Since neoplasms, especially lymphomas, are particularly common lesions in aging cohorts of BL/6 mice, it is surprising that there was no impact upon the survival curve.

A life-span study and associated biochemical studies on a homozygous knockout of a methionine sulfoxide reductase gene were carried out by investigators in the laboratory of Earl R. Stadtman.[8] Their research found evidence for two such genes and the levels of enzyme activity, while substantially reduced, were variable from tissue to tissue, reflecting the relative expressions of the two loci. The methionines of proteins are highly susceptible to sulfoxidation and thus serve as good markers of oxidative stress. There was, in fact, good evidence for increases in the levels of oxidized proteins in their knockout mice and these mice exhibited hypersensitivity to high concentrations of oxygen. The life spans of the enzymatically deficient mice were statistically diminished as compared to wild-type controls, under both normoxic and hyperoxic conditions. Like most knockout mice, these were developed on a background of 129/SvJ. Much less is known about life-table patterns of strain 129 mice in different environments, in contrast to the large amount of data available for the C56BL/6 strain. It is therefore difficult to evaluate the significance of the rather short life spans reported for the control animals. Nevertheless, the study can be interpreted as providing support for the oxidative damage theory of aging.

TRANSGENIC MICE THAT ARE MORE RESISTANT TO OXIDATIVE DAMAGE

It is much easier to make a machine work less efficiently than it is to make it work better. Hence the special interest in transgenic experiments that produce mice that live longer than controls, assuming that the manipulation does not enhance longevity via an unanticipated caloric restriction. (Controls for food intake were carried out in the two experiments noted above.)

Ting-Ting Huang, Charles Epstein, and their colleagues have conducted a long series of experiments using transgenic mice expressing a genomic fragment of the human *SOD1* gene that can provide moderate and ubiquitous overexpression of the enzyme, just the sort of approach that one would wish for a test of the impact upon life span, as a fundamental process of aging might be expected to have various degrees of impact upon all or most tissues. Such overexpression did not prove sufficient to increase the life spans of their transgenic animals, however.[9] This result is perhaps not surprising, as it is possible that one would require a balanced portfolio of appropriate enzymes, such as catalase and glutathione peroxidase, to deal with downstream products of the overexpressed SOD1. As the authors suggest, increased levels of SOD1 might be beneficial for some tissues or cell types and toxic for others, perhaps depending upon the stage of the life course. In our own unpublished transgenic experiments using a cDNA for human *SOD1* driven by an exceptionally strong promoter and enhancer combination (chick beta actin promoter and CMV enhancer),[10] we could not obtain any viable transgenic animals. We injected at least 957 embryos and obtained 236 pups, none of which carried the SOD1 transgene, clear evidence of toxicity.

Mice homozygous for a knockout of p66[shc], one of three proteins encoded by a mammalian proto-oncogene, were shown to live about one-third longer than controls.[11] These mice were relatively resistant to hydrogen peroxide and ultraviolet light, but not to X-rays, agents that are thought to act, in part, via the generation of reactive oxygen species. These mice were also on a 129SvJ background and the controls had rather short life spans. The cohorts used for the life-span determinations were also relatively small. Moreover, given the evidence that these knockout mice exhibited decreased efficiencies of apoptosis, one might have expected increased incidences of neoplasia, a major cause of death of lab mice. Finally, the colony of mice was infected with the mouse hepatitis virus. Nevertheless, this work was the first to show that a specific mutation can provide substantial increase in the life span of a mouse. It has also led to new lines of investigation that indicate the importance of this work. Of greatest potential significance is the evidence of redox regulation of forkhead proteins via a signaling pathway that is dependent upon the p66 protein,[12] thus making a connection of this mammalian biochemistry with the *daf2, daf16* pathway of *C. elegans* and the related pathways that have been studied in fruit flies and in dwarf mice.[1] The recent observations that p66-deficient mice exhibit reduced vascular cell apoptosis and amelioration of experimentally induced atherosclerosis is also of potential relevance to the pathobiology of human aging.[13]

Junji Yodoi and his colleagues have provided evidence that overexpression of human thioredoxin in transgenic mice may extend life span.[14] A variety of lines of evidence indicate that these mice are protected from oxidative stress, providing important support for the oxidative damage theory of aging.

For several years, my colleagues and I have been attempting to synthesize "antimutator" strains of mice using transgenic methods. Our first experiment (unpublished) attempted to overexpress a cDNA for yeast apurinic endonuclease.[15] We were not successful in increasing the endogenous levels of activity, however, and did not pursue life-span and mutagenesis studies. We next attempted to overexpress cDNA constructs for human *SOD1* (as noted above) and *SOD2*, but failed to obtain viable transgenic pups. Overexpression of a cDNA for human catalase, using the same promoter and enhancer combination (as noted above), was more successful.[16,17] The experimental approach was to direct, in separate experiments, the additional catalase to one of three organelles—the peroxisomes (the physiological locus), nuclei, and mitochondria. The latter result has produced the most interesting findings, including ~19% increases in median life spans as well as increases in maximum life spans of mice overexpressing catalase in mitochondria as compared to litter-mate controls.[21] Particularly strong expressions were noted in heart and skeletal muscle. The current analysis of the pathology indicates a significant amelioration, in the catalase transgenics, of subendocardial fibrosis in old animals. That pathology is reminiscent of what is observed in elderly human subjects with congestive heart failure. The transgenic "MCAT" line appears to be resistant to oxidative stress, as evidenced by protection of mitochondrial aconitase activity and resistance to paraquat. The genetic background is mixed C57BL/6 and C3H, but it will be of interest to cross the transgene to other genetic backgrounds. It will also be of interest to develop animals with conditional expression, variable degrees of expression, and more ubiquitous expression. Crosses with SOD2 overexpressors will also be of interest.

A NEGLECTED EXPERIMENTAL APPROACH

My first love in science was with mammalian somatic cell genetics. When I started work in cell culture more than 40 years ago, progress was impeded by the limited replicative potentials of normal diploid somatic cells. One could not readily carry out replicate plating and serial subcloning with such materials. Research was also hampered by the paucity of genetic markers. All that has changed. The most powerful materials now available are pluripotent embryonic stem cells, which can undergo unlimited rounds of replication whilst maintaining their potential to differentiate into a variety of tissues *in vitro*. For mouse geneticists, the greatest attraction, of course, is that cells selected to express particular phenotypes can be passaged, via chimeras, to the germ line, thus creating colonies of animals for genetic and detailed phenotypic analysis. Our first attempt at using such an experimental paradigm was carried out with a line of multipotent embryonic carcinoma cells to demonstrate a proof of principle: namely that one could select for stem cells that were highly resistant to oxidative stress and show that their differentiated progeny, including neuronal cells, were also resistant to oxidative stress. We used a strategy of serial exposures known to have been effective in other systems in producing regional gene amplifications. We were indeed successful in demonstrating this proof of principle.[18] Our selected stem cells and their derived neuronal cells were indeed oxygen resistant. The stem cells exhibited anti-mutator properties.[18] In unpublished follow-up studies, we were able to create a few chimeric mice with patches of skin consistent with chimerization by differentiated progeny of the oxygen-resistant stem cells selected in the laboratory (FIG. 1). Our hope was that other labs with greater resources would be able to carry out the next steps for this line of research, which would include passage of the engineered cell through the germ line and the positional cloning of the locus or loci responsible for the phenotype, as expressed, for example, in tail fibroblast cultures. The citation index has failed to reveal any evidence of such follow-up!

Other somatic cell approaches could be used with pluripotent embryonic stem cells, including random mutagenesis and various modalities of gene transfer. In theory, at least, one could create, in the laboratory, gene actions that took millions of years to evolve in nature.[19]

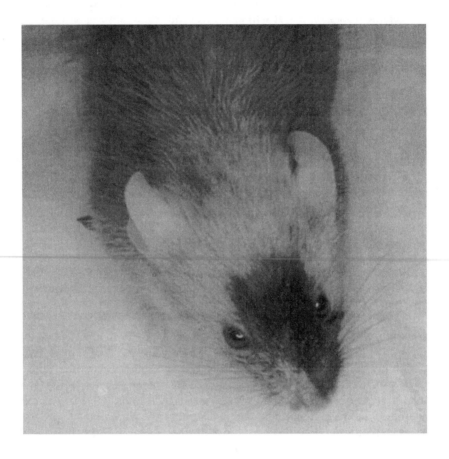

FIGURE 1. A chimeric mouse showing expression of a C57BL/6 phenotype (a patch of black hairs) consistent with the expression of differentiated progeny of a line of pluripotent C57BL/6 stem cells (ES5) selected for resistance to oxidative stress. Cultures of C57BL/6 embryonic stem cells proven to be capable of germ-line transmission[20] were kindly provided by Dr. Carol Ware, Dept. of Comparative Medicine, University of Washington. Mass cultures were challenged by growth in 95% oxygen and surviving clones were pooled and sequentially passaged in 95% oxygen for increasing periods of time (2, 3, 5, and 11 days), after which the emerging, oxygen-resistant cells were utilized in attempts to create chimeric mice via injection of inner cell masses of blastocysts derived from hybrid mouse genotypes. Several hundred attempts yielded only a few such chimeras, probably because of chromosomal lesions in most of the surviving cells. We surmise that less draconian selection schemes would be permissive of a higher efficiency of chimerization and germ-line transmission of the engineered genotype.

REFERENCES

1. PARTRIDGE, L. & D. GEMS. 2002. Mechanisms of ageing: public or private? Nat. Rev. Genet. **3:** 165–175.
2. HARMAN, D. 1956. Aging: a theory based on free radical and radiation chemistry. J. Gerontol. **11:** 298–300.
3. FRIDOVICH, I. 2004. Mitochondria: are they the seat of senescence? Aging Cell. **3:** 13–16.
4. BLOOMFIELD, G. & C. PEARS. 2003. Superoxide signalling required for multicellular development of *Dictyostelium.* J. Cell Sci. **116:** 3387–3397.
5. MACDONALD, D.L., T.L. TERRY, L.B. AGELLON, *et al.* 2003. Administration of tyrosyl radical-oxidized HDL inhibits the development of atherosclerosis in apolipoprotein E-deficient mice. Arterioscler. Thromb. Vasc. Biol. **23:** 1583–1588.
6. VAN REMMEN, H., Y. IKENO, M. HAMILTON, *et al.* 2003. Life-long reduction in MnSOD activity results in increased DNA damage and higher incidence of cancer but does not accelerate aging. Physiol. Genomics **16:** 29–37.
7. LI, Y., T.T. HUANG, E.J. CARLSON, *et al.* 1995. Dilated cardiomyopathy and neonatal lethality in mutant mice lacking manganese superoxide dismutase. Nat. Genet. **11:** 376–381.
8. MOSKOVITZ, J., S. BAR-NOY, W.M. WILLIAMS, *et al.* 2001. Methionine sulfoxide reductase (MsrA) is a regulator of antioxidant defense and lifespan in mammals. Proc. Natl. Acad. Sci. USA. **98:** 12920–12925.
9. HUANG, T.T., E.J. CARLSON, A.M. GILLESPIE, *et al.* 2000. Ubiquitous overexpression of CuZn superoxide dismutase does not extend life span in mice. J. Gerontol. A Biol. Sci. Med. Sci. **55:** B5–9.
10. FUKUCHI, K., M.G. HEARN, S.S. DEEB, *et al.* 1994. Activity assays of nine heterogeneous promoters in neural and other cultured cells. In Vitro Cell Dev. Biol. Anim. **30A:** 300–305.
11. MIGLIACCIO, E., M. GIORGIO, S. MELE, *et al.* 1999. The p66shc adaptor protein controls oxidative stress response and life span in mammals. Nature **402:** 309–313.
12. NEMOTO, S. & T. FINKEL. 2002. Redox regulation of forkhead proteins through a p66shc-dependent signaling pathway. Science **295:** 2450–2452.
13. NAPOLI, C., I. MARTIN-PADURA, F. DE NIGRIS, *et al.* 2003. Deletion of the p66Shc longevity gene reduces systemic and tissue oxidative stress, vascular cell apoptosis, and early atherogenesis in mice fed a high-fat diet. Proc. Natl. Acad. Sci. USA **100:** 2112–2116.
14. MITSUI, A., J. HAMURO, H. NAKAMURA, *et al.* 2002. Overexpression of human thioredoxin in transgenic mice controls oxidative stress and life span. Antioxid. Redox Signal. **4:** 693–696.
15. FUKUCHI, K.I., D.D. KUNKEL, P.A. SCHWARTZKROIN, *et al.* 1994. Overexpression of a C-terminal portion of the beta-amyloid precursor protein in mouse brains by transplantation of transformed neuronal cells. Exp. Neurol. **127:** 253–264.
16. SCHRINER, S.E., A.C. SMITH, N.H. DANG, *et al.* 2000. Overexpression of wild-type and nuclear-targeted catalase modulates resistance to oxidative stress but does not alter spontaneous mutant frequencies at APRT. Mutat. Res. **449:** 21–31.

17. SCHRINER, S.E., C.E. OGBURN, A.C. SMITH, *et al.* 2000. Levels of DNA damage are unaltered in mice overexpressing human catalase in nuclei. Free Radic. Biol. Med. **29:** 664–673.
18. OGBURN, C.E., M.S. TURKER, T.J. KAVANAGH, *et al.* 1994. Oxygen-resistant multipotent embryonic carcinoma cell lines exhibit antimutator phenotypes. Somat. Cell Mol. Genet. **20:** 361–370.
19. LANE, N. 2002. Oxygen, The Molecule that Made the World. Oxford University Press. New York.
20. PESCHON, J.J., D.S. TORRANCE, K.L. STOCKING, *et al.* 1998. TNF receptor-deficient mice reveal divergent roles for p55 and p75 in several models of inflammation. J. Immunol. **160:** 943–952.
21. SCHRINER, S.E., N.J. LINFORD, G.M. MARTIN, *et al.* 2005. Extension of murine life span by overexpression of catalase targeted to mitochondria. Science **308:** 1009–1011. E-publication on May 5, 2005.

Aging and Genome Maintenance

JAN VIJG, RITA A. BUSUTTIL, RUMANA BAHAR, AND
MARTIJN E.T. DOLLÉ

University of Texas Health Science Center, San Antonio, Texas 78245, USA

Geriatric Research Education and Clinical Center, South Texas Veterans Health Care System, San Antonio, Texas 78229, USA

ABSTRACT: Genomic instability in somatic cells has been implicated as a major stochastic mechanism of aging. Using a transgenic mouse model with chromosomally integrated lacZ mutational target genes, we found mutations to accumulate with age at an organ- and tissue-specific rate. Also the spectrum of age-accumulated mutations was found to differ greatly from organ to organ; while initially similar, mutation spectra of different tissues diverged significantly over the lifetime. To explain how genomic instability, which is inherently stochastic, can be a causal factor in aging, it is proposed that randomly induced mutations may adversely affect normal patterns of gene regulation, resulting in a mosaic of cells at various stages on a trajectory of degeneration, eventually resulting in cell death or neoplastic transformation. To directly address this question we demonstrate that it is now possible to analyze single cells, isolated from old and young tissues, for specific alterations in gene expression.

KEYWORDS: genome instability; somatic mutations; gene regulation; aging

INTRODUCTION: SOMATIC MUTATIONS AS A CAUSE OF AGING

Somatic mutagenesis, a stochastic process *par excellence*, has been considered for a long time to be a major causal factor in age-related cellular degeneration and death.[1,2] Mutations—that is, irreversible changes in DNA sequence organization—are inextricably linked to the evolution of different life forms by providing the substrate of natural selection. However, too many mutations, without a mechanism to escape their adverse effects, can be harmful to a cell population. In this respect, mutations are a two-edged sword. In-

Address for correspondence: Professor Jan Vijg, University of Texas Health Science Center, STCBM, 15355 Lambda Drive, Suite 2.200, San Antonio, TX 78245. Voice: 210-562-5027; fax: 210-562-5028.

vijg@uthscsa.edu

Ann. N.Y. Acad. Sci. 1055: 35–47 (2005). © 2005 New York Academy of Sciences.
doi: 10.1196/annals.1323.007

deed, as has been demonstrated in unicellular organisms, mutations decrease fitness and, at least in the absence of sex or recombination, can lead to senescence-like phenomena and population extinction.[3–5] The effect of random mutations on the fitness of a cell population is well illustrated by the work of Elena and Lenski, who compared average fitness (i.e., growth rate) for three groups of *E. coli* strains, harboring one, two, or three randomly introduced insertion mutations. Average fitness was found to decline with the number of mutations.[6]

Populations of *E. coli* cells are not the same as organs and tissues of mammals and an experiment similar to that done by Elena and Lenski is difficult to carry out with mammalian cells in view of their much larger genomes and different genomic organization. Nevertheless, it is conceivable that, similar to relatively small populations of unicellular organisms without the opportunity for sexual reproduction, the somatic cells of multicellular organisms would also be vulnerable to deleterious mutations, which are expected to accumulate over time, eventually resulting in a senescent phenotype. In contrast to unicellular organisms, which represent both germ line and soma, somatic cells of metazoa do not need to maintain genetic variation to provide for evolutionary change. Therefore, in theory, maximization of genome maintenance mechanisms, only for their somatic cells, could prevent any significant mutation accumulation in such organisms. However, evolutionary logic would not predict a further optimization of cellular maintenance and repair than strictly necessary to reach the age of first reproduction.[7] In this context, it is likely that already at reproductive maturity the maximum number of somatic mutations compatible with optimal fitness will have been reached. Even slight increases of the mutation load above this threshold may start to have an adverse impact on the structure and function of an organism. In order to begin testing the hypothesis that mutation accumulation affects fitness in mammals, methods are needed to quantify and characterize spontaneous genomic mutations in different tissues and organs.

First, it is important to distinguish DNA mutations from DNA damage. DNA damage is continually inflicted in cells by such endogenous and exogenous agents as oxygen free radicals and ultraviolet radiation and involves chemical alterations in DNA structure. Such alterations can easily lead to a non-informative or less informative template—that is, a structure that can no longer serve as a substrate for faithful replication or transcription. Since this is a universal problem in cells, highly conserved systems have evolved that are capable of removing or tolerating the damage. In intricate coordination with cell cycle control systems, such DNA damage signaling and repair pathways should ensure genome stability and permit the continuation of processes of transcription, replication, and cell division.[8] When DNA damage levels are too high, cells can activate cellular responses, such as senescence or apoptosis, resulting in permanent cell cycle arrest or cell death, respectively. These and other stress responses are likely to contribute to age-related tissue degeneration and functional decline and could explain some of the observed concerted gene-expressional changes in a tissue during aging.

In contrast to DNA damage, DNA mutations are changes in a DNA sequence that can be transmitted to daughter cells. Hence, mutations are not altering the DNA chemical structure but merely its sequence organization. They can affect a gene, gene-regulatory region, or some non-coding part of the genome. Mutations are usually introduced as a consequence of errors made during replication or repair of a damaged DNA template. Mutations can vary from point mutations, involving single or very few base pairs, to large deletions, insertions, duplications, and inversions. In organisms with multiple chromosomes, DNA from one chromosome can be joined to another and the actual chromosome number can be affected. Because mutations are rare and do not affect DNA chemical structure they are not easy to detect and the total number of mutations in the average cell of an aged tissue cannot be quantified. Hence, while we know that DNA damage induces a variety of cellular responses, the possible impact of its stochastic endpoint (i.e., the spectrum of DNA mutations) on the aging process is unknown.

DETECTING SOMATIC MUTATIONS IN THE AGING MOUSE

In the past, mutation detection *in vivo* has been limited to cytogenetic analysis of actively proliferating cells, such as lymphocytes, for the occurrence of chromosomal aberrations. Later, smaller mutations, such as point mutations, could also be detected in such cells, using selectable marker genes, the most popular being the HPRT locus test.[9] Both cytogenetic tests and the HPRT assay have indicated the accumulation of mutations with age in lymphocytes from both humans and mice.[10–13] However, these results have been interpreted with caution in view of the fact that the assays used could only be applied to actively proliferating cells. This may offer a poor reflection of the *in vivo* system, where the majority of adult human and animal cells only rarely undergo cell division. In order to extend these studies to the *in vivo* situation, we have developed transgenic mouse models harboring chromosomally integrated bacterial mutation reporter genes, which can be recovered from their integrated state, transferred to *E. coli,* and then analyzed for mutations. One of these models, based on chromosomally integrated plasmids containing the lacZ reporter gene (FIG. 1), has made it possible to quantify and characterize a wide range of somatic mutations (including large genome rearrangements) at a neutral, non-expressed marker locus in various mouse organs and tissues as the animals age.[14,15] Using these mice we have demonstrated that mutations at the lacZ locus accumulate with age in most organs and tissues, albeit at greatly different rates (FIG. 2).[16,17]

Organ specificity is also present in the mutational spectra of the lacZ gene *in vivo*. Mutations in the lacZ reporter mouse model can be characterized by

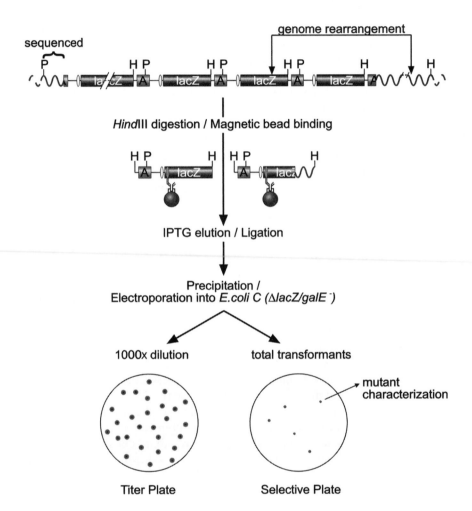

FIGURE 1. Schematic depiction of the LacZ-plasmid model for mutation analysis. In this system, plasmids are rescued by excision of genomic DNA with HindIII, followed by their separation from the mouse genomic DNA using magnetic beads, precoated with a lacI repressor protein. The plasmids are then ligated and transferred to *Escherichia coli* C (ΔlacZ, galE⁻) using electrotransformation. A small amount of transformants is plated in medium with X-gal to determine the total number of plasmids rescued. The remainder is plated on the lactose analogue p-gal, to select only the cells harboring a mutant lacZ gene. The mutation frequency is the ratio of the colonies on the selective plate versus the colonies on the titer plate (times the dilution factor).

restriction digestion and/or sequencing of the positively selected lacZ-mutant plasmids recovered from a mouse tissue (FIG. 1). Mutations that do not alter the restriction pattern are point mutations, that is, single base changes or very small deletions. Mutations that cause changes in the restriction pattern are deletions and other types of rearrangements. Most of this latter type of mutation involves genome rearrangements, with one breakpoint in a lacZ gene of the plasmid cluster and one breakpoint elsewhere in the mouse genome. Physical characterization of 49 genome rearrangement mutations, mainly from heart and liver of young and old mice, indicated intrachromosomal deletions or inversions, varying from smaller than 100 kb to 66 Mb, as well as translocation events.[18]

While initially, at young age, the mutation spectra were more or less the same for all organs, they started to diverge significantly during aging. While, for example, in heart and liver both point mutations and genome rearrangements were found to accumulate, in small intestine the age-related increase was entirely due to point mutations.[16] In old but not in young animals, point-mutational spectra were found to differ greatly between postmitotic organs and more proliferative tissue. While we observed a high frequency of G:C to A:T base pair substitutions at CpG sites in brain and heart, a much more varied pattern was seen in liver, spleen, and small intestine.[19]

FUNCTIONAL IMPACT OF RANDOM MUTATIONS

An important question raised by the results obtained with the lacZ reporter mouse involves the functional impact of the observed mutation load and its increase with age. For most organs the age-related increase was small (i.e., about 2-fold on average), while in brain and testes virtually no increase was observed (FIG. 2). (Unpublished results from our laboratory suggest intra-organ variation in mutation accumulation; for example, while in the brain as a whole no increase was observed, both hypothalamus and hippocampus did show an about 2-fold increase in mutation frequency with age.) While the functional properties of an aging organ can become compromised, even if most of the cells still function optimally (for a discussion of the potential importance of small, upstream changes in aging, see Kirkwood *et al.*[20]), it is difficult to see how a relatively small number of random mutations can adversely affect a genome with about 30,000 protein-coding genes, which represent no more than about 2% of its entire sequence. The chance that one of these random mutations will affect a gene would appear to be very small.

A relatively simple organism, such as *E. coli,* has about 4,000 protein-coding genes constituting almost 90% of its total sequence. Humans and mice have realized their increased structural and functional complexity not by dramatically increasing the number of their protein-coding genes but merely by increasing the size and diversity of their transcriptomes. In humans and mice

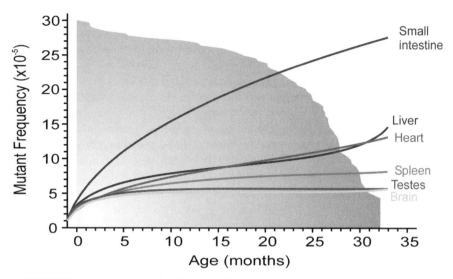

FIGURE 2. Spontaneous lacZ mutant frequencies of various tissues in transgenic lacZ-plasmid line 60 mice. The *gray* fading area represents the survival curve of the lacZ-plasmid transgenic mice, which is not different from normal control mice of the same strain (for further details, see Vijg and Dollé[33]).

almost half of the genome is transcribed.[21] It is assumed that this non-coding transcribed part of the genome has a regulatory role, which is greatly facilitated by the unique single-stranded nature of RNA. Therefore, while only few spontaneous mutations are likely to hit protein-coding genes, at least half of the spontaneous mutation load of an aging mammalian cell would be expected to occur in gene-regulatory regions. Even a relatively small number of mutations could therefore exert some adverse effect on the cell.

A second potential mechanism by which random mutations could influence patterns of gene regulation is through gene dose effects or position effects of regulatory sequence interactions. As mentioned above, a substantial fraction of spontaneous mutations accumulating in old tissues such as heart are genome rearrangements (e.g., deletions, inversions, and translocations). These mutations, which can involve millions of base pairs (see above) most likely find their origin in errors during double-strand break repair. They can be expected to result in partial haploidization of genomic regions or the loss of spatial interactions between regulatory sequences and promoter regions. This could lead to variations in gene expression. Due to their size, even at a very low absolute number, the effects of such mutations could be profound.

Hence, random mutations are much more likely to affect genome function in mammals than previously suspected, in view of the large fraction of their genome that now appears to be relevant for transcriptional control. The real impact would ultimately depend on the total number of mutations and the mutation spectrum, which is likely to differ from cell type to cell type (see above). According to our calculations, the total mutation load per diploid cell in liver would increase from about 60 mutations (about 10 of which are large genome rearrangements) in a young mouse to about 200 mutations (about 30 rearrangements) in an old mouse. These estimates are based on mutation frequencies at the 3-kb lacZ gene of about 3×10^{-5} in young animals to about 10×10^{-5} in old mice.[18] These spontaneous mutation frequencies are in good agreement with results obtained by others, using another, somewhat smaller reporter locus in mice[22] or the HPRT assay on splenocytes.[23] The real mutation load *in vivo* is likely to be even higher than these estimates, owing to the occurrence of mutational hotspots. For example, we previously reported spontaneous somatic and germ line mutation frequencies in a lacZ transgenic mouse model, with the reporter integrated near the pseudoautosomal region of the X-chromosome, that were up to hundred times higher than the average lacZ transgenic line.[24] Notoriously unstable loci, such as simple tandem repeats, can show mutation frequencies in somatic tissue of the mouse as high as 7%.[25] The functional relevance of such mutational hotspots is unclear, but it is conceivable that they contribute to a general destabilization of the genome during aging.

Any functional effect of a mutation in a gene-regulatory region would be enormously enhanced through epistatic effects. For example, it has recently been demonstrated that haploinsufficiency of the Nkx3.1 locus in the mouse increases the probability of stochastic activation or inactivation of its target genes.[26] The results of this study, which involved more than 50 Nkx3.1 target genes in the mouse prostate, revealed a spectrum of dosage sensitivity, varying from relative insensitivity to Nkx3.1 dosage to complete loss of expression even in the Nkx3.1 heterozygotes.

The functional impact of the alterations in the activity of functional pathways that may result from genomic mutations is likely to be cell type- and tissue-dependent, in the context of individual genetic make-up and environmental conditions. Each tissue or cell type has a unique set of active functional modules (groups of proteins that work together to execute a function), the activity of which is primarily determined by transcriptional regulation of the genes involved, with individual genetic, environmental, and lifestyle factors as modifiers. As shown above, mutations accumulate with age in a tissue-specific manner, possibly as a function of their utilization of genome maintenance systems. Gradual mutation accumulation in an aging tissue affecting patterns of gene regulation in a stochastic manner would result in a mosaic of cells, varying from cells that escaped significant damage, to cells with severe dysfunctions, transformed cells, and cells that are dying.

The stochastic effect of mutation accumulation on the fitness of individual cells through random alterations in gene expression is schematically depicted in FIGURE 3. Although gene expression is generally understood as coming

Age-related stochastic loss of function

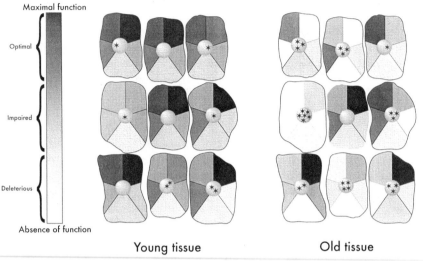

Young tissue   Old tissue

＊ Mutation

FIGURE 3. Model for the stochastic effect of spontaneous mutations on cell function. Each color compartment symbolizes a given function, as determined by the corrected relative expression of a certain number of genes. Random mutations result in loss of transcriptional control, which will affect different cellular functions in a random manner. This results in increased heterogeneity of the cell population with more cells suffering from severe loss of function.

from a sample sometimes representing millions of cells, the concept of an average cell fails to account for the mosaic behavior that is probably a major characteristic of age-related cellular degeneration and death. To some extent variable gene activity can be expected, even in tissues of young, healthy individuals, due to either intrinsic noise, stochastically inherent to normal gene expression, and extrinsic noise, due to fluctuations in cellular components or in the local milieu.[27] The latter could be offset by such factors as redundancy between genes, integration of expression over time or relatively stable protein levels.[28] However, in tissues of old individuals it is conceivable that random molecular alterations, such as the random accumulation of genomic alterations predicted by our results with the lacZ reporter locus, will cause severe expression changes, the physiological effects of which can no longer be dampened by functional overlap or posttranscriptional controls.

If the scenario described above is correct, one would expect increased cell-to-cell variation in gene expression as a function of age. To test this hypothesis, we are presently studying expression levels of multiple genes in individual cells directly taken from their young or old tissue environment. For this purpose, a quantitative, unbiased procedure to amplify global mRNA from single cells is essential. We used the method reported by Klein *et al.*,[29] using a single poly-dC primer, making all amplified sequences equally GC-rich and allowing a high annealing temperature. The method was applied to single cardiomyocytes, enzymatically dissociated from old and young mouse hearts. To verify the reliability of the amplification method in maintaining correct

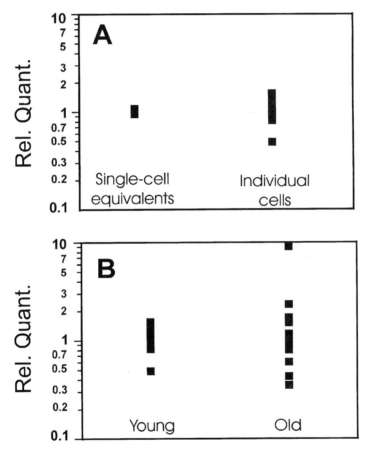

FIGURE 4. Relative quantitative evaluation of the expression level of β-actin versus GAPDH by real-time PCR. In panel **A**, a comparison was made between 10 single cell equivalents (10 replicate global mRNA amplifications of the equivalent of a single cell taken from a pool of several hundred lysed cardiomyocytes; *left*)) and 15 single cardiomyocytes from the heart of a young mouse, each deposited in a tube and subjected to global mRNA amplifications (*right*). Panel **B** shows that there is increased cell-to-cell variation in the relative expression level of β-actin or GAPDH in heart of a 27-month-old mouse as compared to the heart of a 6-month-old mouse. Results are expressed as $\Delta\Delta C_T$, linearized and plotted on a log scale.

gene-to-gene representation in individual mRNA levels, we repeatedly amplified the equivalent of a single cell from a pool of lysed cardiomyocytes. The results indicate an experimental error in the same range as the experimental error of the real-time PCR assay used to assess gene expression levels (in this case β-actin versus GAPDH; FIG. 4A, left). By contrast, β-actin gene expression in single cells showed significant variation (FIG. 4A, right). Interestingly, when comparing 15 cells from a 6-month-old mouse with 15 cells from a 27-month-old mouse, the cell-to-cell variation was significantly higher among the old cells (FIG. 4B). While these results need to be confirmed for other genes and other tissues, they suggest that individual cells vary in the relative abundance of expression of a single gene and that this variation increases with age.

FUTURE PROSPECTS

Aging can be defined operationally as a time-dependent loss of fitness that begins to manifest after the organism attains its maximum reproductive competence. Assuming that aging is not the result of a pre-programmed set of events, as now seems clear, but instead a consequence of a natural limitation in repairing damage in its informational macromolecules, programmed and stochastic mechanisms are no longer mutually exclusive explanations for the remarkable consistency in cellular degeneration and death within and across species. Ever since the discovery of DNA repair as a key mechanism for balancing mutation rates between the need for evolutionary change and optimal cellular fitness, aging has been considered as the result of genomic instability.[30] This "somatic mutation hypothesis of aging" seamlessly connected with the demonstration that human progeroid syndromes, such as Werner's syndrome and Cockayne syndrome, discovered a century ago, were almost all caused by a heritable defect in a DNA repair gene. Similar findings with mouse DNA repair mutants confirm the important role of genome maintenance in retarding aging.[31] The recent discovery, first in nematodes and fruit flies but then also in mice, of survival pathways, alterations in which can increase or decrease life span, possibly by manipulating cellular defense systems such as DNA repair and antioxidant defense, confirms the concept of aging as a continuous attempt to retard an inevitable onslaught of damage.[32] What are the pathophysiological endpoints of damage accumulation?

First, it is likely that cellular responses to damage, such as the activation of cell senescence and cell death pathways, are a major cause of aging phenotypes, such as organ atrophy. This would appear to be a pre-programmed cause of aging, since it is a consistent response of a sizable fraction of the cell population. However, cellular responses to damage are unlikely to be the only explanation for aging, since even very old organisms still appear to have ample tissue capacity left to function optimally.

Stochastic mechanisms, such as the accumulation of random mutations, would be expected to yield subtle changes in gene-transcriptional regulation. The accumulation of such changes could explain a variety of aging phenotypes. For example, haploinsufficiency at tumorigenic loci, due to the kind of large deletion mutations observed in old mice (see above), would be expected to influence expression of multiple target loci and result in pre-neoplastic lesions. Similarly, random genetic alterations could lead to subtle alterations in insulin sensitivity and glucose metabolism, causing late-onset diabetes. Both genetic (the genotype as present in the zygote) and environmental factors would be major determinants of the onset of such aging-related disease phenotypes.

Altogether, the concept presented here suggests a mechanism to explain how a stochastic process such as mutation accumulation can have functional consequences for cell populations organized in tissues and organs. Owing to the recent emergence of increasingly sensitive techniques to study individual cells for alterations in genome organization and gene expression, various aspects of this stochastic concept of aging are now testable. This is demonstrated by the example shown in FIGURE 4, but other single-cell assays at the level of genomic changes are available or under development in various laboratories.[29]

ACKNOWLEDGMENTS

This research was supported by NIA program project AG17242.

REFERENCES

1. SZILARD, L. 1959. On the nature of the aging process. Proc. Natl. Acad. Sci. USA **45:** 30–45.
2. FAILLA, G. 1958. The aging process and carcinogenesis. Ann. N.Y. Acad. Sci. **71:** 1124–1135.
3. KIBOTA, T.T. & M. LYNCH. 1996. Estimate of the genomic mutation rate deleterious to overall fitness in *E. coli.* Nature **381:** 694–696.
4. ANDERSSON, D.I. & D. HUGHES. 1996. Muller's ratchet decreases fitness of a DNA-based microbe. Proc. Natl. Acad. Sci. USA **93:** 906–907.
5. BELL, G. 1988. Sex and Death in Protozoa. Cambridge University Press. Cambridge, UK.
6. ELENA, S.F. & R.E. LENSKI. 1997. Test of synergistic interactions among deleterious mutations in bacteria. Nature **390:** 395–398.
7. KIRKWOOD, T.B. & S.N. AUSTAD. 2000. Why do we age? Nature **408:** 233–238.
8. HOEIJMAKERS, J.H. 2001. Genome maintenance mechanisms for preventing cancer. Nature **411:** 366–374.

9. ALBERTINI, R.J. 2001. HPRT mutations in humans: biomarkers for mechanistic studies. Mutat Res. **489:** 1–16.
10. RAMSEY, M.J. *et al.* 1995. The effects of age and lifestyle factors on the accumulation of cytogenetic damage as measured by chromosome painting. Mutat. Res. **338:** 95-106.
11. TUCKER, J.D. *et al.* 1999. Frequency of spontaneous chromosome aberrations in mice: effects of age. Mutat. Res. **425:** 135–141.
12. DEMPSEY, J.L., M. PFEIFFER & A.A. MORLEY. 1993. Effect of dietary restriction on in vivo somatic mutation in mice. Mutat. Res. **291:** 141–145.
13. JONES, I.M. *et al.* 1995. Impact of age and environment on somatic mutation at the hprt gene of T lymphocytes in humans. Mutat. Res. **338:** 129–139.
14. BOERRIGTER, M.E. *et al.* 1995. Plasmid-based transgenic mouse model for studying in vivo mutations. Nature **377:** 657–659.
15. DOLLÉ, M.E. *et al.* 1996. Evaluation of a plasmid-based transgenic mouse model for detecting in vivo mutations. Mutagenesis **11:** 111–118.
16. DOLLÉ, M.E., *et al.* 2000. Distinct spectra of somatic mutations accumulated with age in mouse heart and small intestine. Proc. Natl. Acad. Sci. USA **97:** 8403–8408.
17. DOLLÉ, M.E. *et al.* 1997. Rapid accumulation of genome rearrangements in liver but not in brain of old mice. Nat. Genet. **17:** 431–434.
18. DOLLÉ, M.E. & J. VIJG. 2002. Genome dynamics in aging mice. Genome Res. **12:** 1732–1738.
19. DOLLÉ, M. E. *et al.* 2002. Mutational fingerprints of aging. Nucleic Acids Res. **30:** 545–549.
20. KIRKWOOD, T.B. *et al.* 2003. Towards an e-biology of ageing: integrating theory and data. Nat. Rev. Mol. Cell Biol. **4:** 243–249.
21. SHABALINA, S.A. & N.A. SPIRIDONOV. 2004. The mammalian transcriptome and the function of non-coding DNA sequences. Genome Biol. **5:** 105.
22. HILL, K.A. *et al.* 2004. Spontaneous mutation in Big Blue mice from fetus to old age: tissue-specific time courses of mutation frequency but similar mutation types. Environ. Mol. Mutagen. **43:** 110–120.
23. ODAGIRI, Y. *et al.* 1998. Accelerated accumulation of somatic mutations in the senescence-accelerated mouse. Nat. Genet. **19:** 116–117.
24. GOSSEN, J.A. *et al.* 1991. High somatic mutation frequencies in a LacZ transgene integrated on the mouse X-chromosome. Mutat. Res. **250:** 423–429.
25. YAUK, C.L. *et al.* 2002. A novel single molecule analysis of spontaneous and radiation-induced mutation at a mouse tandem repeat locus. Mutat. Res. **500:** 147–156.
26. MAGEE, J.A., S.A. ABDULKADIR & J. MILBRANDT. 2003. Haploinsufficiency at the Nkx3.1 locus: a paradigm for stochastic, dosage-sensitive gene regulation during tumor initiation. Cancer Cell **3:** 273–283.
27. ELOWITZ, M.B. *et al.* 2002. Stochastic gene expression in a single cell. Science **297:** 1183–1186.
28. LEVSKY, J.M. & R.H. SINGER. 2003. Gene expression and the myth of the average cell. Trends Cell Biol. **13:** 4–6.
29. KLEIN, C.A. *et al.* 2002. Combined transcriptome and genome analysis of single micrometastatic cells. Nat. Biotechnol. **20:** 387–392.
30. STREHLER, B. L. 1995. Deletional mutations are the basic cause of aging: historical perspectives. Mutat. Res. **338**: 3-17.

31. HASTY, P. *et al.* 2003. Aging and genome maintenance: lessons from the mouse? Science **299:** 1355–1359.
32. KIRKWOOD, T.B. 2003. Genes that shape the course of ageing. Trends Endocrinol. Metab. **14:** 345–347.
33. VIJG, J. & M.E. DOLLÉ. 2002. Large genome rearrangements as a primary cause of aging. Mech. Ageing Dev. **123:** 907–915.

The Use of Genetic SNPs as New Diagnostic Markers in Preventive Medicine

CHARLES R. CANTOR

SEQUENOM, Inc., San Diego, California, USA

ABSTRACT: Using an automated mass spectrometric genotyping platform, we have completed more than ten whole-genome SNP scans on phenotypically stratified population pools. The pools are usually constructed to represent one ethnicity, one gender, and one phenotype, classified as strictly as possible. From 28,000 to 91,000 different SNPs are used for each study, and the pools typically contain DNA from 300 different individuals. Significant correlations between SNP allele and phenotype are first reproduced in the pools, then replicated on individual DNA samples (deconvolution of the pools), and then where possible replicated in completely independent populations.

KEYWORDS: SNPs; human disease genes; schizophrenia; breast cancer; cardiovascular disease; new genetic medicine

After completion of the human genome sequence, human genetics has changed remarkably. It is now possible to find the genes that underlie complex disease, reasonably efficiently and reasonably inexpensively. It appears that on the order of 40 genes will be found to play a major role in an average complex disease. Many other genes will be minor modifiers, but for diseases such as diabetes, breast cancer, or schizophrenia, an average of 40 genes will be found to have a small but finite contribution - a number small enough to render them possible to locate.

Unfortunately, our understanding of quantitative traits based on as few as 3, 4, or 5 genes is minimal. By comparison, a 40-gene disorder is fairly complicated.

At the start of this article, to demonstrate our current capabilities, I will discuss two diseases not especially involved with aging: schizophrenia and breast cancer. I will conclude with the results of a very unconventional study

Address for correspondence: Charles Cantor, 3595 John Hopkins Court, San Diego, CA 92121 USA. Voice: 1-858-202-9012; fax: 1-858-202-9020.
ccantor@sequenom.com

Ann. N.Y. Acad. Sci. 1055: 48–57 (2005). © 2005 New York Academy of Sciences.
doi: 10.1196/annals.1323.009

inspired by the phenomenon of human aging, which may have significant impact for cardiovascular disease.

THE CHALLENGE OF FINDING GENES

How do we know whether human traits are inherited or dominated by the environment? We can study monozygotic twins, who have identical DNA. Any pattern of variations present in the DNA of one twin is present in the DNA of the other. (This is not true of dizygotic twins, who are essentially only half genetically identical, like any other siblings.) If we compare the concordance of properties in identical twins and fraternal twins, we can make a quantitative estimate of the degree to which any particular property is dominated by the genes or by the environment.

Many thousands of twins have been phenotyped extensively. Heritability is defined on a 0-to-1 scale; a heritability value of 1 (which never occurs among humans) means that genetics is totally dominant, while heritability of 0 (which also never occurs among humans) means that there is no heritability. Most heritability values in humans are around 50/50, which means simply that genetics among humans is about a 50% effect.

Because it is not acceptable to control human breeding, all human genetics studies are retrospective. They involve surrogate markers, which are presumably functionless DNA variations that reside close to, and co-associate with, a gene involved in the trait under study.We look for linkage disequilibrium between a surrogate marker and a functional single nucleotide polymorphism (SNP) or other meaningful genetic variation nearby.

How to define the term "nearby" in the context of the human genome is the source of much confusion. In family studies, the patterns over which the genome is conserved extend tens of millions of bases. You can scan across 10% of a chromosome, and cover the genome with 1,000 markers, which is relatively simple. Unfortunately, family studies have not worked well for complex human traits, because human families are not big enough to generate meaningful statistical power. Many researchers have turned instead to founder populations, such as those in Iceland, Newfoundland, and Finland, where the patterns of conservation extend over about a million bases.

Interesting genes have been found in such founder populations, but it is not straightforward to generalize from one founder population to the rest of humanity. Often, unfortunately, published associations based on the population in Iceland have not been reproduced in studies of gene databases in the United States, Northern Europe, and Australia.

What would be ideal would be whole-genome case-control association studies. In Caucasians, genetic patterns in the out-bred population extend (are conserved) over regions about the size of a gene (25,000 bases). Covering the entire genome in a search for linkages would require 100,000 gene-associated markers. Before the human genome was sequenced, such a number was unattainable. Today it is relatively straightforward to find 100,000 gene-associated markers, allowing us to navigate through the genome at will, at least in the case of Caucasians.

Unfortunately, in people of African descent, conserved regions are much smaller, extending only around 5,000 bases rather than 25,000. Sadly, that factor of five is significant, and human genetics remains expensive for black populations.

There are four requirements to find genes that underlie complex disease: well-phenotyped populations, because poor phenotypes are misleading; a dense set of gene-associated genetic markers, because of the aforementioned practical limitations inherent in studying genes among human beings; a technology platform with an intrinsic error rate below 3–5%, because the effects we are looking for are very small; and a trick, because most methods that biologists use are too costly.

Using traditional human genetics to locate genes contributing to complex major diseases would require examining 500 to 1,000 people for 25,000 to 100,000 genetic markers—upwards of 100,000,000 measurements. This is not feasible. But we have discovered, and others have confirmed, the feasibility of studying genetics in human DNA pools, rather than among individuals. Using DNA from 300 people in a phenotypic class, we make equal molar mixtures of DNA to create pools representing cases and controls. The average genotype of these two pools is the allele frequency.

The sacrifice in doing this is the inability to distinguish between heterozygotes and homozygotes, losing some statistical power. The advantages are shrinking the cost of the study and also the amount of DNA (and therefore blood) required from each individual. Genetic studies that would have cost $50,000,000 two years ago (and therefore were not carried out) cost less than $500,000 to do today (and are therefore feasible).

SEQUENOM'S METHODS FOR LOCATING
SNP GENETIC MARKERS

We carry out a first pass case–control comparison, usually with a set of 28,000 top-quality SNPs. These generate some associations, which we reproduce. Later we deconvolute the pools and carry out individual genotyping, setting the statistical thresholds to derive 50 candidate genes from every study. As in any data-intense study, most of these will be false positives. Approximately 10% are true positives. The challenge is to distinguish the true positives from the false positives.

A set of 28,000 SNPs is less than the aforementioned number of 100,000 needed for full coverage of the genome, so we know that we will miss at least half of the real genes. On the other hand, we can expect to find at best up to half of the genes that are responsible for each complex trait.

The SNPs we have used result from a collaboration between SEQUENOM and GlaxoSmithKline. Starting with 250,000 putative genetic markers, we produced 100,000 valid markers that are polymorphic and uniquely mapped. These are all in the public domain. Our studies involve subsets of these markers.

In the past 18 months, we have completed whole-genome surveys for 12 case–control studies, most of them using our set of 28,000 high-quality SNPs. Most of these were traditional case–control designs, involving approximately 300 cases and 300 controls. We tripled the number of markers for studies of Type II diabetes and lung cancer, but this did not triple the results.

With the exception of Alzheimer's disease (which we intend but have not yet begun to study), we plan no further case–control studies. We have discovered about 60 genes which we are very confident play a major role in complex disease. We hope others will continue the search, but these are more than we can easily analyze.

DOCUMENTING THE VALIDITY OF RESULTS

Before discussing the genes we have found, it is important to recognize the sad history behind the search for genes that underlie complex human traits. A recent article in *Genetics in Medicine* observed that, of 166 published associations between genes and complex human traits such as schizophrenia and obesity, only six are reproducible.[1] The other 160 presumably represent false positives, generating numerous articles in scientific journals and major daily newspapers that are simply wrong.

Many of these associations were published by authors as the result of a single genetic study. In contrast, we have completed 12 genetic studies, representing more human genetics measurements than in the whole history of the field by all other authors. We can compare measurements between studies, an unprecedented luxury in the field of human genetics. For example, in a genetic study of diabetes we should enrich for genes that by any mode of annotation or interpretation might have something to do with diabetes—obesity, glucose, metabolism, and so on.

The fact that these studies are performed blind (statisticians do not know the identity of the SNPs or even the disease under study) argues that some of these are true positives. As we would have predicted, as well as discovering novel genes that underlie complex disease, we also re-discovered the few that have already been found by other methods.

One of these is a peroxisome proliferator-activated receptor (PPAR).[2] Although the genetic effect of PPAR is very weak, we discovered it in the diabetes scan. In high-density lipoprotein (HDL) we found CETP and lipoprotein lipase; in lung cancer, CD-44; in schizophrenia, dopamine decarboxylase, and so on. In the case of melanoma, we found a germ-line predisposition to the disease in the gene for B-Raf kinase. Somewhat later, two papers were published showing somatic gain-of-function mutations in the same gene in malignant melanoma and in pre-cancerous moles.

Sometimes we locate genes that fall in linkage regions, or loss-of-heterozygosity regions, which have been reproduced by others who could not identify the gene because of the large size of the region. For example, a high-density SNP scan in lung cancer showed an extraordinarily high concentration of hits at one end of a known loss-of-heterozygosity region. We now know which gene involved in lung cancer is located there.

When we show a SNP that is strongly associated with a disease, we go back and sequence the DNA in this region from 100 individuals, find all the SNPs in that region, and then carry out multiple-locus association studies to narrow in on the particular gene and verify that we have found a real positive linkage, rather than a mere fluctuation. Given the troubled history of molecular human genetics, the onus of proof must be on geneticists to prove that each of their discoveries is a true positive, not a false positive.

There are three means of accomplishing this. The gold standard is to repeat the genetic association in a truly independent population. Identical results in multiple independent studies document a real association, but if the results in the multiple populations are not the same, the explanation is unclear. Genetic heterogeneity or different environmental effects in the multiple populations could be responsible. Or the first finding could be a false positive. In such a case, we try a fourth population, or more.

A second possibility, if the gene looks very interesting, is to try to validate the results *in vitro* or in model organisms, in an attempt to generate phenotypes consistent with the disease in question. Alternatively, one may find additional associations in human studies, either with a drug already known to be efficacious in the disease in question, or with a secondary phenotype that, added to specific clinical information, can act as an independent statistical validation.

In a typical case–control study we find four or five genes, roughly 10% of the 40 that we estimate are involved in any major multi-gene disorder. For some of the genes implicated in Type II diabetes, we have as many as four independent replications of associations with SNPs, and we are confident that these are true positives.

A GENE FOR A SECONDARY PHENOTYPE

One example of a convincing result from the study of a single population is schizophrenia, for which there is very strong secondary phenotype. We were able to obtain access to members of a very interesting population of subjects, all of whom were taking olanzapine, currently the major prescribed drug for schizophrenia. These subjects must have had at least a moderate response, because the side-effects of olanzapine are so significant that it is discontinued in any patients who do not respond to the medication. In this study we had no access to side-effect data, but we did have access to drug-response information. We had some additional secondary phenotype information; we knew which of the individuals had hallucinations, delusions, both or neither. We performed a whole-genome scan on this population. We were able to correlate not just case controls with schizophrenia, but we also were able to subtype, with interesting results.

The gene identified in these studies is a peptide carrier, a very well-known protein that has not been subjected to much study in the brain. Upon close scrutiny, we learned that from the case–control data that the association was limited to individuals who had been diagnosed with schizophrenia clinically, but who were not having either active hallucinations nor active delusions. Stratifying the population in this way, we obtained P values approaching those found in the association between the APOE-4 haplotype and Alzheimer's disease. In this case we have not identified a gene for schizophrenia, but one that determines a secondary phenotype.

We also have three genes that show fairly good correlation with schizophrenia, but also a fairly good P value correlating with the level of response identical to olanzapine. One of these genes codes for a neurotransmitter. We intend to try to confirm these findings by reproducing these studies in an independent population.

A GENE NOT PREVIOUSLY LINKED WITH DISEASE

In studies comparing two or more populations, it is important to be certain of the "independence" of the populations. In the case of breast cancer, we have replicated our results in separate populations in Germany and Australia. Because there is relatively little genetic admixture in both Germany and Australia, one can be relatively unconcerned about genetic artifacts in comparing the two populations.

One of the genes we have uncovered in these populations is in the Herceptin-signaling pathway, but a different gene than the well-known transcriptional repressor. We have studied the expression of this gene in five different breast cancer cell lines with different phenotypes, some of which are estrogen-responsive, and others of which are not. In the case of the well-known and actively studied transcriptional repressor in the Herceptin pathway, which is being explored as a potential drug target for breast-cancer chemotherapy, the deleterious form is a loss-of-function mutation. Therapy involving this gene would require an agonist, and it is not clear how to create an agonist for a transcription factor. The deleterious form of the gene we have found, in contrast, is a gain-of-function mutation, which may be possible to inhibit.

The gene in question is not as highly expressed in breast cancer tissues as the more well-known transcription factor. However, an alternative splice variant, which is expressed at very low levels in breast-cancer cell lines, almost completely halts proliferation of the cells if it is downregulated by RNA interference. Attempts to suppress the normal transcript, however, have no effect whatever.

Looking in more detail, we find that suppressing this alternative splice variant has the effect of stopping growth and eventually killing the cells. Classical tests show that they have been driven into apoptosis by siRNA (small interference RNA). By now we have a considerable understanding of how this gene acts within the Herceptin pathway. Unfortunately, as a transcription factor, it is unlikely to be a drug target.

Another gene we have implicated in breast cancer, however, is more likely to be suitable for drug development. It a nucleotide exchange factor which loads and unloads GTP and GDP into G-proteins, and thus can modulate G-protein signaling pathways.

In both the German and Australian populations, there is a substantial increase in the frequency of this allele among breast cancer patients, compared to controls. In homozygotes for the allele, the association is larger. The P-values are almost identical in the two populations, and the odds ratios for increased risk of breast cancer are almost identical.

Previous to these studies, the gene in question was not suspected of involvement in breast cancer. It is highly expressed in four of our five breast-cancer cell lines, but is not expressed in normal breasts or in any other normal tissue, with the exception of a slight expression in brain.

In two cell lines, RNA interference of this gene suppresses growth by about 50% under normal culture conditions. But if cells are grown on Matrigel at low serum concentrations, the siRNA stops growth very effectively, as compared with a non-functional siRNA control.

Attempting to associate the nucleotide exchange factor with a more specific phenotype, we used a model system from metastasis, a Boyden chamber, in which cells are seeded on one side of a porous membrane, which divides a chamber with a low serum concentration from one with a high serum concentration. Metastatic cells are able to cross the membrane by chemotaxis to reach the higher-serum solution.

We found that among breast cells in which siRNA had suppressed the nucleotide exchange factor, the ability to cross the membrane is essentially eliminated, while control cells cross the membrane *en masse.* Thus we believe we have found a useful target for a drug that may be able to suppress metastasis in breast cancer. Classical transfection tests classify this as an oncogene. Cells such as NIH-3T3 transfected with this gene become immortalized and grow into colonies.

THE POWER OF GENETICS OVER GENOMICS

The conclusion from all of our studies is that if you collect a case–control population, and are willing to spend upwards of $500,000, you will find on average 5 genes that play a major role in complex disease. Over the next few years, we can anticipate the discovery of genes that are major players in most major diseases.

This is the power of genetics over genomics. Probably every single gene in the genome, manipulated it in the right way, could be used to produce a disease. But the human population has not yet existed long enough as a species to experience all of the harm that of our genes can do. In reality, only a very small number of our genes as yet are bad actors. The final section of this article deals with an extremely bad actor that we are beginning to understand.

This study was designed and executed by Andreas Braun, our chief medical officer, who carried out all of the studies discussed above. In this case, he decided to test the hypothesis that, because young people do not develop the major complex, adult-onset diseases, a major risk factor in complex disease is age.[2] Braun reasoned that, if we collected a large healthy population and stratified it by age, any genetic variations which have a massive impact on the health or survival of people should decline in prevalence as a function of age, because the people who possess those genes have dropped out of the healthy population by becoming sick or dying.

We chose to define the term "healthy" by using voluntary blood donors, mostly in Bakersfield, California, because these individuals are healthy enough to volunteer and to make their way to blood donation centers, where they are accepted as blood donors. We have very little phenotypic information about these individuals.

About 5 or 10 genes have emerged from of this study. In most cases we have not followed up because we have no idea what disease is involved. In one case, where we were able to take an educated guess, the gene is called *D-AKAP2,* which codes for dual-specificity A kinase-anchoring protein 2. What the protein AKAP2 does is to bind protein kinase-A and position it in cells. The D stands for dual function, because it binds multiple isoforms of protein kinase-A which have different effects.

We were fortunate to find a coding polymorphism in linkage disequilibrium with this gene, in which an isoleucine is the protective or neutral allele and a valine is the deleterious allele. We found this gene originally in Caucasians, defining young as under 40 and old as above 60. There is a dramatic drop in the prevalence of the deleterious allele as a function of age, almost a factor of two in homozygotes. We see the same effect in women, in men, and in Hispanics. This one deleterious allele seems to be responsible for removing roughly 8% of people from the healthy population in our study. This is a gigantic effect, but it does not reveal which disease is involved.

Susan Taylor, the discoverer of this gene, recognized that our polymorphism represents the protein's binding site for protein kinase A.[3] D-AKAP2 is a very large protein, whose coding sequence is otherwise 100% conserved between human and mouse. The polymorphism is in the region that binds protein kinase-A (PKA). Because there were suggestions that proteins in this family could be involved in cardiovascular disease or obesity, we took a sample of several thousand twins in the UK, for whom we had some cardiovascular parameters, and examined their DNA for associations involving this polymorphism. We found that individuals who have the deleterious genotype at this polymorphism (GG) also have a minor EKG irregularity. Intervals in both the QRS mean and the PR mean are shortened. These are not outside the normal range, but they would be significant enough to stop administration of a drug in a clinical trial.

In biochemical studies, the deleterious allele increases the affinity of the D-AKAP2 for the RI isoform of protein kinase-A by a factor of 3 or 4. It is a small effect that has dramatic consequences inside the cell.[4] Both alleles target the RI isoform to mitochondria; the normal or protective allele does so only slightly for RI but the deleterious allele targets the RI isoform to mitochondria excessively.

To address why this would be deleterious, we used site-directed recombination to create allele-specific knock-in mice. Three of the strains are homozygotes; a fourth seems to be a homozygous lethal. Three of these are single-site amino acid changes, and the fourth is a 3-site amino acid change. One should exaggerate the human deleterious phenotype. The second one probably would have very little effect. The third one might be healthier. The fourth one, we would predict, would tremendously exaggerate the deleterious human phenotype.

We have characterized these mice for various cardiovascular parameters. Morphologically, we see no striking effects, but electrocardiograms of these mutants show three kinds of abnormalities. We see ventricular premature beats, supraventricular premature beats, and supraventricular tachycardia. According to cardiologists, ventricular premature beats are often fatal. The mutant we expected to have deleterious effects is the one that shows the ventricular premature beats. It is also the one that shows most of the supraventricular beats and the one that shows the tachycardia. The genetically normal mice are normal.

Thus it appears that *D-AKAP2,* a single gene, has a large enough impact on health to be isolated from what was basically a huge public health survey. Perhaps there are a few more such single-gene "bad actors" in the human genome. Given time, we can find them.

REFERENCES

1. HIRSCHHORN, J.N., K. LOHMUELLER, E. BYRNE & K. HIRSCHHORN. 2002. A comprehensive review of genetic association studies. Genet. Med. **4:** 45–61.
2. ALTSHULER, D., J.N. HIRSCHHORN, M. KLANNEMARK, *et al.* 2000. The common PPARγ Pro12Ala polymorphism is associated with decreased risk of type 2 diabetes. Nat. Genet. **26:** 76–80.
3. KAMERER, S., L. BURNS-HUMURO, Y. MA, *et al.* 2003. Amino acid variant in the kinase binding domain of dual-specific A kinase anchoring protein 2: a disease susceptibility polymorphism. Proc. Natl. Acad. Sci. USA **100:** 4066–4071.
4. BURNS-HAMURO, L., Y. MA, S. KAMERER, *et al.* 2003. Designing isoform-specific peptide disruptors of protein kinase A localization. Proc. Nat. Acad. Sci. USA**100:** 4072–4077.

Longevity Determinant Genes: What is the Evidence? What's the Importance?

Panel Discussion

RICHARD CUTLER, *Moderator*

L.P. GUARANTE, THOMAS W. KENSLER, FRED NAFTOLIN, DEAN P. JONES, CHARLES R. CANTOR, GEORGE M. MARTIN, *Panelists*

RICHARD CUTLER: An idea I had for many years is the general concept that there might be specific genes that are important to govern an aging rate. That is, in spite of the vast complexity of the aging process itself, there may be a few key genes that play an important role in governing how fast the aging process itself takes place. Some data generated over the last few years seems to be consistent with the idea. But of course there is still a lot more work to be done. One of the questions is, how do we stand with that hypothesis? Of course, it would be great if it was true, because it would indicate it may not be too complicated to increase the expression of a few genes, like thyrodoxin genes or the expression of an ARE complex that really may play an important role. Of course, it won't work at all if oxidative stress is not playing a key role. That's one of the things we are certainly interested in discussing, and is probably going to be a common theme in many of the meetings in the future.

QUESTION: The more I kept thinking about what Dr. Guarante said about SIR2 and the promise of intervention, the more I wanted to return to the dichotomy between nutritional inputs and pharmacologic interventions. The case is well made that oxidized NAD is signaling the system that the flow of electrons is not as vigorous, presumably, which allows a little bit of NAD to accumulate and go ahead and do the signaling. Whereas if you are eating a lot of food and electrons are continually pouring in, then the carbon is going to cholesterol and fatty acids, and the electrons are going to oxygen and superoxide and hydrogen peroxide, all things you don't really want. That's where the pharmacologist intervenes to affect SIR2. But what's going to affect the appetite that brought all that carbon and electrons into the liver? You might get SIR2 going, but then the liver is going to make a lot of cholesterol, fatty acids and superoxide.

LEONARD P. GUARANTE: What will be the effect if you don't restrict calories, if you elicit the genetic response to calorie restriction? We really don't

Ann. N.Y. Acad. Sci. 1055: 58–63 (2005). © 2005 New York Academy of Sciences.
doi: 10.1196/annals.1323.010

know, but it will be an issue. A very good point. Biology is not a theoretical science, its an empirical science. You perform experiments and see the results. In the simple systems, a modest upregulation of SIR2 is a good thing, but if you raise the levels of SIR2 too high in yeast, it becomes disadvantageous, so there's clearly an optimum. With any drug, of course, dosing is really important, and it could be that we are going to have to get the level just right, but if SIR-2 is really affecting these various pathways, for example fat mobilization and utilization, you'll be able to keep eating and the fat is going to be cleared.

COMMENT: You still either have to either burn it off or you store it — one or the other. If you are burning it off eating all these calories, and not exercising, you will have the same obesity problem America is faced with now.

GUARANTE: We definitely have a mechanism to burn fat. We burn it in liver and muscle. Mice with the insulin receptor knocked out in the fat cells are very lean, but they eat a lot. They eat more than the control littermates. They are burning the fat and living long. Your comment is very important and I don't have the answer, but I don't think there will necessarily be a problem.

RICHARD CUTLER: I'd just like to inject a question here. One of the things we are interested in is comparing human with chimpanzee to ask what is unique about human genetics that allows us to live twice as long as the chimp. What is striking to me is that the human model doesn't look like the caloric restriction model of the chimpanzee. The glucose level is the same — we don't have particularly less fat than the chimp, and maybe we have more fat, but we still live substantially longer. What is the difference in SIR-2 expression,and does this model work in mice but not in humans.?

GUARANTE: We won't know whether calorie restriction really would extend life span in humans for a long time. I think a study is now going on asking whether the physiological changes that accompany calorie restriction occur in humans with the same kind of kinetics as they occur in other systems. I think that will be a gauge as to whether it's likely to work, and if those changes happen — reduction in insulin, body temperature, glucose, so on — I would say that's a good omen. Actual studies are going to be brutally difficult, and it would be a very cruel irony if after years of trials, life span were not extended.

QUESTION: I'd like to direct this question to Dr. Kensler. The number of genes upregulated by D3T is fairly substantial, as I recall: more than 200. There are many proteins that depend for their biological activity on their conformation, and thus the potential target of intramolecular disulfide interchange, polymerization, is very real. Several hormones depend on disulfides for proper conformation, among them insulin, growth hormone, and prolactin. I am curious whether antioxidant response elements have been identified in tissues where those hormones are produced. Have the hormones themselves, or their biological activity, been looked for in any of the models you described?

THOMAS W. KENSLER: I'm not sure I can give you a cogent answer. The simple answer is no.Some research is just beginning to be developed about cross-talk between different signaling pathways, including some of the nuclear orphan receptor pathways in NRF-2, and ARE responsive genes.

CHARLES CANTOR: I can't resist adding a comment. The problem of false positives that I alluded to in genetic studies is equally true in gene-expression studies, and most of those upregulated or downregulated genes are false-positives in everybody's studies, until they have been reproduced in multiple populations.

FRED NAFTOLIN: I really loved the talk about SIR-1, and since you always hurt the ones you love, I have to ask you this question: It has to do with whether we think of aging as living to 100 as a natural process, or living to 40 at reproduction as the natural process, and then whatever you get after that is icing on the cake. We can talk about burning off those extra calories, but the fact is that 70-year old people don't do enough exercise to burn off those extra calories. When we have these discussions, we always have to preface them by saying that we have never lived this long. The centenarians we heard about were born at a time when public health measures and antibiotics had not doubled our average life span. They are not *a priori* a good example of us, because they made it through a strainer that existed around 1900 and 1920 that doesn't even exist any more. People don't die of childbirth, or infection, or hemorrhage, or accidents at the rate that they did at that time. They are different people. The rest of us have achieved 50 years of life that we have not been evolved to have. How are we going to deal with the fact that we are post-reproductive, therefore without adaptation, being dunked into the pool with 50 more years to go and all we have is a repertoire that we learned when we were 1 to 50?

RICHARD CUTLER: It's an error to think that after a person reaches sexual maturity there's no more selection. There is a factor of function in primate longevity; the longer-lived the primates, the more they depend on learned behavior versus instinctive behavior. A lot of that goes into teaching your children and progeny. An argument can be made that, particularly for humans and these other animals who have a high dependence on learned behavior, there is certainly a very important evolutionary role: post-reproductive competency. The other thing we are asking is, if we can understand what is unique about the genetics and biochemistry of centenarians, can we apply that early enough in our lives so that we can live a younger, healthier life span? It's well known that for most of human history the average life span was about 25 years. Very few people lived much past 50, but we generally believe that the genetic potential for longevity was always there. The problem was with those saber-toothed tigers and everything around them. The main point here is, what can we do now to try to change our genetics, or intake, and maybe the pharmacology, to live a few more years younger longer?

QUESTION: Tell me what you are doing differently that may extend the time until you meet your demise?

DEAN P. JONES: I lecture to first-year medical students on nutrition at the end of our biochemistry course. I have actually thought this through quite a bit, talking to them about what they will say in the future to patients. Also I do three types of exercise: a resistance exercise, a cardiovascular exercise, and just simply walking. I try to get in half an hour to 40 minutes of walking every day. I also pay attention to nutrition, having three balanced not-exces- sive- calorie meals a day. It's hard work to come up with three balanced meals a day—but it's of greatest importance.

RICHARD CUTLER: I'm probably one of the worst examples. My difficulty is that I don't have much wrong with me, so I haven't been doing much of anything. Just a few days ago I went through the Kronos Optimal Health Pro- gram, in which they put you through every kind of test you can think of, and then you talk to a nutritionist and an exercise person. They said, "Dr. Cutler, you're going to have to start doing the right thing." Of all people, I probably should have done this years ago, but I'm not going to wait for a problem. I'm going to get into this exercise program at last. The big motivator I have now is the wife. She says, I just can't stand looking at you. That motivates too.

QUESTION: My question, perhaps naively, stems from the concept of old science versus new science. A few years ago, all the buzz was about telomer- es. I was a little surprised not to hear a word about them yet. Dr. Cantor, could you comment about the status of that research?

CHARLES CANTOR: I'm not the right person to comment, but telomeres are important.

GEORGE M. MARTIN: Richard Cawthon of the University of Utah pub- lished a paper in which he had assessed the telopmeric lengths of banked pe- ripheral blood leukocytes and he made correlations with the health and life span of members of pedigrees from Utah. He found surprisingly good evi- dence that those with shorter teleomeres, on average, were more likely to die at an earlier age from two causes: infectious diseases, which makes sense, as he was studying cells involved in the immune response and cardiovascular disease, which was interesting as it invokes proliferative aspects of the patho- genesis. His work has therefore rejuvenated interest in the relationship of te- lomere biology and atherogenesis. Oxidative damage may in fact be a mechanism that leads to shortened telomeres; it's on the list of possibilities. It's simply a correlation, not a cause, but it's interesting and deserves confir- mation and extension.

QUESTION: A very brief comment and then a question for the panel. The brief comment is for the gentleman who said something about how hard it is to get 75-year-olds up off the couch. I would encourage you to come to Sun Valley, where the average 75-year-old is either cross-country or downhill ski- ing every day, and is incredibly bright and active. My question concerns world aging. No one has mentioned that the highest concentrations of centenarians in the world are the in the province of Bama in China, the mountains of Peru and the island of Okinawa. How valid is it to compare our population with others to discern differences in lifestyle? Has this longevity in these areas been over a duration of time or is it only recent?

RICHARD CUTLER: Unfortunately, Thomas Perls is not here. That would be a great question for him. Does anyone here on the panel want to respond to that?

GEORGE M. MARTIN: There was a poster at the meeting of the Gerontological Society of America this year by a group that had been following the Okinawan population—one of the three you mentioned. There are recent secular changes in diet that are quite dramatic. These translated into dramatically increased heights in the current Okinawan baby boomers. There has been atremendous increase in caloric intake in that population. There are already some demographic trends suggesting that they are not living quite as long. We'll see how that plays out. I don't know about the authenticity of the data on centenarians in the two other places you mentioned. There have been some retractions of claims of excessive longevity in some populations. It's hard to document the authenticity of the long lives in those remote places.

PANEL MEMBER: There is a point to be made in those centenarian studies, It is very important to make sure that you can establish the real age of these people, because many of them actually lie. They like to be thought of as very old when they really are not. It's very difficult to authenticate the ages in centenarians.

QUESTION/COMMENT: Does anybody on the panel take any multivitamins and if so, do they break it down into individual ones, like vitamin C and vitamin E? More important, the comment: When I see my 70 and 80 year old patients, they seem to be very happy and contented. Stress, I think, is a major factor in why we are not very healthy. The young people of today are so stressed out. They want more. They strive to do a lot more than they can really do. Whereas older people were more content and exercised and had time to enjoy the simple facts of life.

RICHARD CUTLER: I think everyone recognizes the importance of vitamins. The real necessity to take a vitamin, of course, is in the second world countries, where clearly they are having a problem with malnutrition. Here in the United States, I don't think it's that much of a problem.

QUESTION: I want to return to the dichotomy in our society between nutrition and pharmacology or nutriceuticals. The idea of our modern food chain, or food web, has been to narrow the genetic diversity of the raw materials and to funnel the marketing through a very limited number of major international organizations; this decreases our options. We are moving to highly refined encapsulated essence of something and leaving out the fiber. One of the main characteristics of the last 100 years of North American diets is the removal of fiber. In fact, in the late 19th century, Post and Kellogg discovered fiber and tried to make a lot of money from their cereals. You can still get All Bran. The question is, even if you have found the key essence of some single chemical that might save our lives, one of the things we are still faced with is eating enough vegetables to provide enough fiber to satiate appetite. Satiety and appetite control remain one of the topics not addressed today. Appetite is probably the worse enemy of the North American people right now. I'm wondering what is your advice to all the Americans who are not eating five vegetables a day now?

PANEL MEMBER: You raised a very good point about the homogenization of the American diet and food supply. I'm not trying to come up with an alternative food substance, but something that would serve as a supplement to what is otherwise a well-balanced diet. By selecting for these cultivars of a cruciferous vegetable, we can enrich materials that have protective properties. That plant doesn't recapitulate all of our dietary needs and doesn't substitute for many of the other factors that you talked about, such as fiber. We cannot take the reductionist view that a pharmaceutical or a pill or specifically engineered or otherwise selected food materials are going to solve all our problems. We must maintain the broader view that there are many elements of our diet that are beneficial, and we must use our knowledge to better select those foods that compensate for deficiencies or provide some benefit in the form of a supplementation.

QUESTION: I appreciate your sharing your personal secrets to longevity, but I was very surprised that no one is taking an aspirin a day, or a statin. Any comments?

GEORGE M. MARTIN: I can comment. All my cardiology colleagues in the city of Seattle are taking statins. Maybe it hasn't permeated to the pathologists as yet. There is a little evidence of increased risk of hemorrhagic types of stroke. The one thing I don't want is a stroke — I don't mind going out with a coronary occlusion, But I will have to reassess that decision periodically. It's the reason I don't take, or haven't been taking, aspirin. Probably, as a public health measure, it's a pretty good idea. Occasionally there's a colleague who goes to the hospital with bleeding from gastric mucosa, possibly related, in part, from the use of aspirin, perhaps too much aspirin.

RICHARD CUTLER: I think you'll find on a survey here, that most people in this room are probably on a well-defined supplement, statins or whatever. We take reasonably good care of ourselves — except for me, of course.)

Decoding the Pyramid: A Systems-Biological Approach to Nutrigenomics

JIM KAPUT

Laboratory of High Speed Computing and Information, University of California at Davis, Davis, California, USA

ABSTRACT: Nutritional genomics, or nutrigenomics, seeks to understand the effects of diet on an individual's genes and health. Nutrigenomics is a systems-biological science that can be explained by five principal tenets: (1) improper diets in some individuals and under some conditions are risk factors for chronic diseases; (2) common dietary chemicals alter gene expression and/or genome structure; (3) the influence of diet on health depends upon an individual's genetic makeup; (4) some genes or their normal common variants are regulated by diet, which may play a role in chronic diseases; and (5) dietary interventions based upon knowledge of nutritional requirements, nutritional status, and genotype can be used to develop individualized nutrition plans that optimize health and prevent or mitigate chronic diseases. Optimal nutrition may also influence the aging process.

KEYWORDS: nutrigenomics; nutritional genomics; genotype–diet interactions; quantitative trait loci; diet

INTRODUCTION

Biological organisms evolve and adapt to specific environments defined primarily by available nutrients. That is, the DNA in their genomes is selected on the basis of available "metabolizable" chemicals. Although nutrients were generally thought to provide only energy for metabolism, certain chemicals influence an organism's response and adaptation to its environment. The interaction of an organism's genome with its environment defines a set of interactions that can be analyzed at the molecular and genetic level. The details of these interactions may differ between members of a species

Address for correspondence: Jim Kaput, Ph.D, Laboratory of High Speed Computing and Informatics, NCMHD Center of Excellence in Nutritional Genomics, University of California, Davis. One Shields Avenue, Davis, CA 95616, and NutraGenomics, 2201 West Campbell Park Drive, Chicago, IL 60612. Voice: 312-829-3036.
jkaput@ucdavis.edu

Ann. N.Y. Acad. Sci. 1055: 64–79 (2005). © 2005 New York Academy of Sciences.
doi: 10.1196/annals.1323.011

within an environment because each member of the species has seemingly inconsequential variations in its DNA and those gene variants alter its response to its environment. Evolution may be seen in one sense as the selection of organisms best able to utilize and respond positively to nutrients in their environments.

The interface between the nutritional environment and cellular/genetic processes is referred to as nutritional genomics, or nutrigenomics. As a field of science, nutrigenomics seeks to understand the effects of a diet on the activity of an individual's genes and health.[21] This definition of nutrigenomics embodies the disciplines of nutritional science, molecular biology, and, when applied to an individual, genetics and genomics. Since unbalanced diets alter the equilibrium between health and disease, nutrigenomics research also addresses physiology and pathology. Nutritional genomics is, therefore, a systems-biology science, since it analyzes and integrates physiological measurements (such as HDL, LDL, cholesterol, height, weight, enzyme activities, protein levels, metabolite concentrations, etc.) and genotype as measured by expression analyses or more typically by single nucleotide polymorphisms (SNPs or gene variants).

The field of nutritional genomics is better explained as a set of principles:[21]

- Improper diets in some individuals and under some conditions are risk factors for chronic diseases;

- Common dietary chemicals alter gene expression and/or genome structure;

- The influence of diet on health depends upon an individual's genetic makeup;

- Some genes or their normal common variants are regulated by diet and may play a role in chronic diseases; and

- Dietary interventions based upon knowledge of nutritional requirements, nutritional status, and genotype can be use to develop individualized nutrition that optimizes health and prevents or mitigates chronic diseases. Optimal nutrition may also influence the aging process.

EPIDEMIOLOGIC AND PHYSIOLOGIC STUDIES LINK CERTAIN DIETS WITH DISEASE

Deficiencies in nutrients have long been known to affect health. For example, beriberi and scurvy are alleviated by vitamins B and C. Although nutrient deficiencies are largely restricted to individuals in socioeconomically depressed societies, and in particular in post-colonial countries, the consumption of excess calories or specific dietary chemicals also causes disease. Epidemiologic studies have linked unbalanced diets with obesity, diabetes, cardiovascular disease, and certain types of cancer, as well as other chronic diseases.[39,40] These linkages are based upon a statistical association of exposure (in this case, intake of certain nutrients) with incidence or severity of disease in a population. Dietary recommendations, as shown in guides such as the food pyramid, are based upon these statistical associations for a population.

Well-controlled statistical associations have limitations. First, individuals within a population are genetically different and may require more or less of a given nutrient for optimal health (reviewed in Kaput[20]). Analyzing genetic differences among individuals is a key component of nutritional genomics research. Second, associations do not provide information about the mechanisms by which a dietary chemical affects health or disease. Knowing the molecular mechanism is the first step in understanding how to alter nutrient intake to improve health. Nevertheless, epidemiological studies provide valuable information about which nutrients to study at the molecular and genetic levels.

Analyzing nutrient–gene interactions is challenging because of the chemical complexity of food. Corn oil, which may be considered a "simple" processed nutrient source from one plant, has measurable amounts of 9 fatty acids, 9 sterols, more than 12 fatty acid sterols, 5 different tocols, and 12 varieties of triglycerides (TABLE 1). Oils processed from different plants, for example soy or coconut, have different concentrations of the same chemicals and in some cases different chemicals and/or classes. The choice of oil for experiments is usually based upon its known characteristics; for instance, coconut oil is used for studies of saturated fats and corn oil for studies of polyunsaturated fats. However, changing lipid macronutrients will also alter the concentration of "minor" constituents that may have an impact on health. An illustration of this issue is beta-sitosterol, which is found at ~ 0.5 gr/100g

TABLE 1. Composition of corn oil[a]

Fatty Acids (approx. 96 g/100 g corn oil)	Percentage of Total Fatty Acids
C16:0	10.9
C18:0	2.0
C18:1	24.9
C18:2	60.4
C18:3	0.9
C20:0	0.4
C20:1	0.2
C22:0	0.1
C24:0	0.2

TABLE 1. (Continued) Composition of corn oil[a]

Fatty Acids (approx. 96 g/100 g corn oil)	Percentage of Total Fatty Acids
Sterols	**mg/100g**
Campesterol	150.6
Stigmasterol	44.8
β-Sitosterol	496.3
Obtusifoliol	7.8
Unknown A	25.4
Cycloartenol	22.4
24-Methylene cycloartanol	5.9
Unknown B	10.8
Unknown C	7.8
Fatty Acid Sterols	**mg/100g**
Campesteryl palmitate	5.5
β-Sitosteryl palmitate	22.0
Cycloartenyl palmitate	14.9
24-Methylene cycloartanol palmitate	8.9
Campesteryl oleate	17.0
Campesteryl linoleate	26.1
Stigmasteryl linoleate	17.4
β-Sitosteryl oleate	31.4
β-Sitosteryl linoleate	106.3
Cycloartenyl oleate	11.2
Cycloartenyl linoleate	30.6
24-Methylene cycloartanol linoleate	13.8
Other	293.9
Tocols	**ppm**
α-tocopherol	252
β-tocopherol	Trace
γ-tocopherol	774
δ-tocopherol	38
γ-tocotrienol	14
Triglyceride	
13 varieties	

[a]Analyses performed by L. Romanczyk, M&M Mars, Inc., using standard chemical analyses. From Kaput and Rodrigues[21] by permission.

a) Relative Affinities for Estrogen Receptorβ

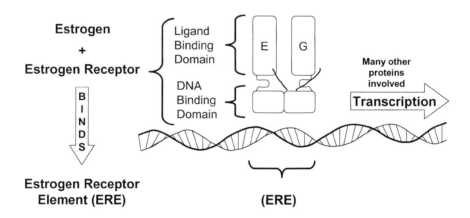

	ERα	ERβ
Estradiol	1	1
Genistein	1×10^{-4}	3.2×10^{-2}

b) Receptors & Expression

FIGURE 1. Certain dietary chemicals activate gene transcription. (**a**) Relative affinities of endogenous (estradiol) and exogenous (genestein) ligands for estrogen receptor α (ER-α) and estrogen receptor β (ER-β). The relative affinity of estradiol is 1, and genestein binds ER-α and ER-β with less affinity. (Adapted from Gutendorf and Westendorf.[16] (**b**) Receptors and expression. Exogenous (G = genistein) or endogenous (E = estradiol) chemicals bind to receptors in the ligand binding domain causing dimerization and binding to response elements in DNA. Transcription of receptor-regulated genes is initiation in conjunction with a host of other transcription factors and coactivators.

of oil in corn, but at 0.15g/100g and 0.04g/100g in soy and coconut oils, respectively. It competes for cholesterol uptake in the intestine, but it also undergoes conversion by gut microflora to androstenedione,[33] a precursor to estrogen. Others have proposed that local production of estrogen is a risk factor for breast cancer.[3] The other biological implication of this example is that what might benefit heart health may increase risks of other diseases.

DIETARY CHEMICALS AND GENE EXPRESSION

Although many dietary chemicals are metabolized to CO_2 and water, producing energy for life, some of the chemicals in diets alter gene expression directly or indirectly. The phytoestrogen genistein is an example of how a nutrient can have a direct effect on gene expression. Gustafsson and coworkers co-crystallized genistein and the estrogen receptor beta (ER-β),[23] a transcription factor that regulates a subset of estrogen-responsive genes. The crystal structure demonstrated that genistein binds in the active site where the endogeneous ligand, estradiol, binds. Although genistein binds with less affinity than estradiol to ER-β (FIGURE 1A), it nevertheless would activate the receptor, causing dimerization, binding to ER-responsive promoters, and initiation of transcription (FIGURE 1B). Other dietary chemicals, such as hyperforin, a chemical found in St. John's wort, have been shown to activate specific transcription factors.[38] One of these transcription factors, the pregnane X receptor, regulates cytochrome P450 genes involved in metabolizing xenobiotics found in plants. This is another example of co-evolution of plants and animals. Many modern drugs, particularly those that are oxidatively metabolized, are substrates for these same P450 enzymes.[26] Some transcriptional ligands are produced by metabolism from nutrients: Certain lipids are converted to eiconosoids that bind to lipid sensors (TABLE 2) such as the retinoid X receptors or PPARs. These lipid-sensor receptors or transcription factors regulate genes that metabolize lipid nutrients. An additional 15–20 other transcription factors are known on the basis of sequence homologies, but their endogenous or dietary ligands have not yet been found.

Other dietary chemicals affect metabolism by affecting signal transduction pathways. Green tea contains the polyphenol 11-epigallocatechin-3-gallate (EGCG), which inhibits tyrosine phosphorylation of the Her-2/neu receptor and epidermal growth factor receptor.[31] This signal-transduction pathway ultimately reduces activity of NF-kβ[7] involved in cancer and inflammatory processes. Docosohexonoic acid (DHA), α-linolenic, linoleic, and oleic acids (among others) affect signal-transduction pathways by altering the activity of GPR40 in a dose-dependent manner.[17] This membrane protein regulates Ca^{2+} flux. These lipids are examples of dietary compounds that indirectly affect gene expression. Many of these processes occur on a short response time, on

TABLE 2. Nuclear receptors and dietary ligands[a]

Regulation[b]	Receptor	Type	Endogenous Ligand	Dietary Ligand
Endocrine	Estrogen	ERα	17β-estradiol	Genistein (4)
		ERβ	17β-estradiol	Genistein (87)
Hormonal lipids	Progesterone		Progesterone	
K_d = 0.01–10 nM	Androgen		Testosterone	and
	Androgen		5α-dyhydro-testosterone	
Feedback paradigm	Mineralocorticoid		Aldosterone	Endogenous metabolism
	Glucocorticoid		Cortisol	Cholesterol precursor
Mixed paradigm	Retinoic acid	RARα	All-*trans* retinoic acid	Vitamin A
		RARβ	All-*trans* retinoic acid	Vitamin A
		RARγ	All-*trans* retinoic acid	Vitamin A
	Thyroid	TRα		Iodine
		TRβ		Iodine
	Vitamin D		1,25-dihydroxy-vitamin D	Vitamin D/sunshine
	Ecdysone		Cholesterol derivatives	Cholesterol
Lipid sensors	Retinoid X		*cis*-9 retinoic acid	Docohexa-enoic acid
	PPAR	PPARα	FA	Pristinic/phytanic
		PPARγ	FA/eicosanoids	Pristinic/phytanic
		PPARδ	?	
Dietary	Pregnane X		Estrogen	Hyperforin
K_d > 1–10 μM			Progesterone	Genistein
			Pregnenlone	Coumesterol
	Liver X		Oxysterols	Cholesterol metabolites
Feedforward paradigm	Farnosoid X		Bile acids	
	Constitutive androstane		Androstenol	Androstenol
			Androstanol	
	Aryl hydrocarbon		?	Indolo3,2-β–carbazole

[a]Information for this table was consolidated from information in Refs. 5, 6. 8, 14, 18, and 21 by permission.
[b]Designation from Chawla *et al.*[5]

the order of hours, but long-term or frequent exposure to the same chemicals may ultimately produce long-term changes in physiological processes.

This summary of how diet affects gene expression underscores the importance of monitoring, controlling, and testing dietary variables when conducting studies in model organisms and humans. Many molecular and genetic studies fail to control for or test for nutrient intake, which may best be summarized as "the diet disconnect." This need to add diet as a variable in experimental design applies not only to basic research, but also to diagnostic and drug development, where diet might alter response to drugs or treatments.[20]

THE INFLUENCE OF GENETIC MAKEUP ON DIETARY RESPONSES

The USDA's food-guide pyramid was designed to provide minimum dietary intakes for the majority of individuals in a population. However, it typically is interpreted as being the optimum diet for everyone. This would assume that all individuals are culturally, socio-economically, physiologically, and genetically identical (see Pagel[27]). Human populations are divided into about 7,000 different languages, a measure of the large number of different cultures.[27] Genetically, humans are more homogenous, differing by only 3 million base pairs out of a total of 3 billion base pairs. This 0.1% difference is responsible for differences in height and weight potential, but also in susceptibility to diseases, including those influenced by diet.

Genetic diversity adds statistical noise to studies of diet in humans; individuals differ genetically in small but significant ways from all other humans. Variations in promoters or in the proteins that regulate transcription will produce variations in gene expression, and, in some cases, physiology. Naturally occurring dietary chemicals will interact with the same classes of proteins in each individual, but because individuals will have different variants of these proteins, the responses between individuals may differ.

One of the best examples of genotype–diet interactions is lactose intolerance. Most mammals do not drink milk as adults, yet about 95% of individuals of Northern European descent have the ability to use this nutrient source.[9] Lactose tolerance arose when a series of mutations occurred about 9,000 years ago in one or more individuals in Northern Europe. Mutations in the promoter of the lactase gene altered the regulation of the gene[37] so that it could be expressed after weaning. The altered regulation provided a selective advantage because milk from humans or domesticated animals is a good nutrient source.[1] Studies of these ancestral mutations, identified as single nucleotide polymorphisms (SNPs), show that individuals with some genetic connection to Northern Europeans have an increased chance of encoding the variants, and therefore are lactose tolerant. It is likely that variants in other genes that metabolize nutrients will be found in populations from different geographic areas of the world, since all animals evolve in response to food availability.[1]

Regardless of the single gene variant one inherits, a single gene cannot predict the response to most nutrients. Any given nutrient is likely to be transported across the intestinal lining and from the intestine to a specific organ or organs by multiple transporters. In addition, nutrients may also be metabolized at any point during this process. Variants in all of the genes in the pathway from absorption to final destination or metabolic fate will affect nutrient availability. The study of the genes and their variants and how they affect physiology and health is influenced by the overall genetic makeup of an individual; that is, the sum of all gene variants in the transport and metabolic pathways contributes to nutrient use in each individual. These pathways, and the genes that encode the enzymes and proteins, are embedded in an overall genetic makeup that also differs among individuals and groups of individuals.

Since humans migrated to all regions of earth over the past 200,000 years,[35]individuals from different geographical regions may respond differently to diets. The rapid increase in obesity and Type 2 diabetes mellitus attests to the effect of genetic background on nutrient metabolism. Although all ethnic groups are affected, individuals with "thrifty genotypes"—that is, genotypes that more efficiently utilize nutrients[4,19,24]—are more susceptible to excess dietary fat and calories. Thrifty genotypes are typically associated with post-colonial regions of the world but also include Native Americans.

CERTAIN DIET-REGULATED GENES ARE INVOLVED IN DISEASE PROCESSES

Laboratory animals provide a useful model to examine genetic differences that lead to different responses to diets. Inbred mice result from brother–sister matings over 20 generations; all mice in the inbred strain are genetically identical (reviewed in Linder[25]). Experiments can therefore be replicated as they cannot among humans, who are genetically unique. Finally, mice are valid model systems for humans because 99% of all human genes[30] are found in mice and disease physiologies are similar among mammals.

Our laboratory developed an experimental strategy to identify genotype–diet interactions using inbred strains of mice fed semi-purified diets in a controlled fashion. In one published study, C57BL/6 and BALB/c mice were fed diets containing 4% or 20% coconut oil or 4% or 20% corn oil for 4 months.[30] Serum triglycerides (TG) and other serum lipids were analyzed. TGs increased in BALB/c mice fed diets with 20% corn oil, but were not significantly affected by increased intake of 20% coconut oil. C57BL/6 mice had the opposite response: corn oil had no effect, but coconut oil caused a significant increase in TGs. Analyses indicated statistically significant interactions be-

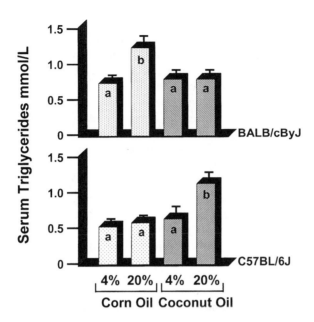

FIGURE 2. Response of triglyceride levels in BALB/c and C57BL/6 mice fed different types and concentrations of dietary fats. Mice were fed balanced diets containing 4% or 20% corn or coconut oil for 4 months. Following a feeding regimen,[29] blood was collected and analyzed by standard methods. Differences in triglycerides were statistically significant, including strain–source (P < 0.0009) and strain–source–level (P < 0.014) interactions. (Adapted from Park *et al.*[29])

tween strain and oil source, and between strain, oil source, and level. These responses are a classic example of genotype–environment interactions. Corn and coconut oils altered the expression of genes that synthesize or metabolize triglycerides, but each strain responded to a different type of oil (FIG. 2).

We used this same comparative-approach model to identify genes that are differentially regulated by genotype (strain A fed diet 1 vs. strain B fed diet 1, and strain A vs. strain B fed diet 2) and diet (diet 1 in strain A vs. diet 2 in strain A, and diet 1 in strain B vs. diet 2 in strain B). Genotype–diet interactions are found when genes are differently regulated by genotype and diet in the comparisons. Genotypes are selected on the basis of their susceptibility to diet-induced disease; for example, strain A would get a diet-induced disease but strain B would be less susceptible to disease on the same induction diet. Gene expression is analyzed before the animals show symptoms of disease, because disease processes themselves alter gene expression. This has been known from studies of cancer dating back to the 1980s.

Our experimental protocol also controls for nutrient status (fed vs. fasted) because the influx of dietary chemicals caused by eating will induce a large number of physiological responses, many of which will alter gene expression.[29,35] Reducing biological and environmental variables is critical for interpreting gene expression data and testing for reproducibility. The experimental design we have developed is also useful for analyzing the effect of dietary supplements or nutraceuticals.

We fed agouti mice (*A/a*) and obese yellow mice (*A^vy^/A*) control diets (100% calories) and 70% calories.[43] Micronutrients, fiber, and vitamins were adjusted to maintain similar intakes in both diets. Agouti and obese yellow mice are genetically identical, except for one gene, which causes overexpression of the agouti protein. The agouti protein is involved in hair color regulation, but also plays a role in the melanocortin pathway involved in weight control (reviewed in Voisey[36]). The *A^vy^/A* mouse weighs up to 65 grams within about 8 months while the *A/a* mouse grows to about 20–25 grams, which is typical of most mouse strains.[41] The overexpression of the agouti protein also causes symptoms of diabetes (hyperinsulinemia, hyperglycemia) and increases susceptibility to cancer in a number of tissues.[42]

Expression profiles of liver mRNA were compared between genotypes fed the same diets and within a genotype fed different diets. Only genes that differed in regulation are of interest, because in order to get a difference in phenotype (in this case, obesity or symptoms of Type 2 diabetes mellitus), gene expression must differ between *A/a* and *A^vy^/A* mice fed the same diets (either 70% calories or 100% calories). This comparative approach identifies genes regulated only by genotypic differences, by diet, and by a combination of diet and genotype.[43] That is, some genes are up- or downregulated only by genotype regardless of the diet, other genes respond to diet regardless of the genotype, and the majority of genes respond to diet based upon genetic makeup. A gene may be regulated by diet in one strain or genotype at a statistically significant level, but not regulated significantly in another strain. To our knowledge, our comparative approach is the only one to identify genes regulated in these different manners at the same time.

Gene expression cannot differentiate cause from effect: diet and genotype may regulate many genes, but only a subset may play a role in changing phenotype from health to disease. The map positions of genes that are differently regulated between genotypes, diets, or by genotype–diet interactions are compared to chromosomal regions known to be associated with disease. These regions are typically determined by quantitative trait loci (QTL) analyses and are public-domain data derived by others. As the name implies, QTL are regions (loci) of chromosomes encoding one or more genes that contribute to a complex trait (reviewed in Brockmann[2] and Flint[11]). This is shown schematically in FIGURE 3. Chromosomal regions marked by dots contribute to Type 2 diabetes mellitus.[15,32,a] Each QTL contributes between 1% and

---

[a]See http://www.informatics.jax.org/searches/marker_form.shtml. Enter QTL for "Type"; under "Symbol/Name" enter diabetes.

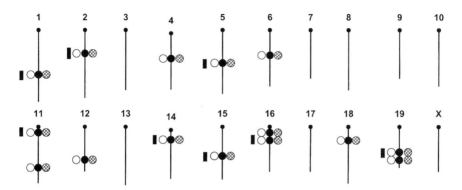

FIGURE 3. Schematic example of quantitative trait loci (QTL) for type 2 diabetes mellitus in mice. T2DM is a complex trait that results from the contribution of many genes, their interactions with each other, and the influence of the environment, including diet, on the activity of the genes. Regions of chromosomes that contribute statistically to incidence and severity of T2DM are marked by circles. Some chromosomes have more than one QTL region (Chr, 11, 16, 19) and others have one. Each QTL contributes different amounts to the overall complex trait, that is, some may be responsible for 1–5% of a specific subphenotype (e.g., insulin levels) and other QTL may contribute more to the trait (e.g., 30 %). T2DM QTLs may be associated with glucose levels, insulin levels, glucose response, or any measurable trait associated with T2DM. QTLs may span 5 to 10 million base pairs and encode many genes, one or more of which contribute different amounts to the complex trait. Genes within the QTL that contribute to the complex trait may be difficult to identify because they may be normally occurring gene variants. However, each gene may have protective alleles, deleterious alleles, or neutral alleles. A subset of QTLs encode genes regulated by diet and involved in producing the complex trait.[20,22,29] Individuals may inherit different combinations of protective, deleterious, or neutral alleles at these QTL, and the mix of alleles is responsible for the range in susceptibility for that individual. Diet contributes to disease incidence and severity by altering expression of the diet-regulated genes at one or more loci. The black boxes near QTL on Chr 1,2,5,11,14,14,16,19 represent loci syntenic with QTL found in humans.[12]

100% to the disease process, but all combined are equal to 100%. The genes at each locus are likely to have alleles that contribute to the disease (deleterious alleles), neutral alleles, or beneficial alleles (FIG. 3). The most severe case would result if deleterious alleles or variants are present at each locus so that the sum total is 100%. Some individuals would have all beneficial alleles and would therefore not develop the disease. Most individuals inherit a mix of deleterious, neutral, and beneficial alleles at different QTLs which explains the differences in genetic susceptibility found in outbred populations such as humans. Some of the QTL identified in different mouse strains have counterparts identified in human QTL studies for the same disease. For example, 8 loci in humans that are associated with diabetes or subtypes of diabetes[12] are syntenic to loci in mice associated with Type 2 diabetes mellitus subphenotypes. Such concordance provides support for using mice as a model for human disease.

Our working hypothesis is that one or more genes at some QTLs are regulated by diet, since unbalanced diets are known to increase the risk and severity of chronic diseases such as obesity and type 2 diabetes. Differentially regulated genes that map within QTL are candidates for contributing to the specific quantitative trait when the diet alters expression of the gene. In lay terms, we are each born with a range of susceptibility based upon the genetic makeup we inherit, but where we fall within that range depends on diet and other environmental variables. Hence, disease susceptibility is not deterministic since a controllable variable (in this case, diet) alters the expression of genetic information and the probability of developing the disease.

Twenty-nine of the genes regulated by diet, genotype, or genotype–diet interactions map to murine diabetic QTL in mice, and 8 of these loci are syntenic (that is, they match) human QTL involved in diabetes.[43] An additional 59 genes mapped to obesity loci. Testing the role of each gene in producing a subphenotype requires additional studies in mice, or association of the genes (or their variants) in humans. A combination of the genes and their variants that we have identified are likely to contribute to diabetes or obesity. Some of these genes are likely to overlap with targets for drugs, while others may be regulated by altering diets specific to the genotype of the individual.

INDIVIDUALIZED NUTRITION

The future promise of nutritional genomics is that, after gene variants are associated with nutrients in the context of genetic makeup, genetic tests will provide information for tailoring diets to each individual. A likely scenario is that diagnostic tests will be done, with the patient under the care of a physician and with the aid and advice of a genetic and nutritional counselor to develop an individualized dietary plan based upon a personal genetic analysis. As society accepts and embraces preventive approaches to health, these tests may be done soon after birth. National and international genetic privacy laws must be enacted before such testing becomes widely available. Society will also have to address a host of consequences of such genetic testing, including the possibilities that insurance companies may offer discounts for "healthy" genotypes and that there may be penalties for individuals who do not follow nutritional advice based upon their genotypes.

Consumer foods also are likely to evolve in tandem with the ability to identify genotypes that respond better or worse to specific food ingredients.[10,13] Although it is unlikely that each individual will have a unique diet (how can food companies produce individual products for each of us?), it is likely that foods may be designed for groups of individuals with similar genotypes.

These groups are not likely to be related to ethnicity, since genetic variation within an ethnic group is larger than that between groups. Individuals within each group may need more or less of specific nutrients such as vitamins, dietary supplements such as herbs, and minerals. Nutrigenomics also offers hope of analyzing how much of a dietary supplement may be optimum for each individual. Optimized diets are likely to maintain health and delay effects of aging and aging-related disorders.

Within nutritional genomics, research efforts are currently being applied to the study of chronic diseases such as obesity, cardiovascular diseases, and Type 2 diabetes mellitus. These diseases are associated with food abundance and high caloric intake in affluent, industrialized countries. Since a large proportion of the world's population still suffers from malnutrition, the emphasis on studies of these diseases has been disparaged. However, because the research strategies and methods of nutritional genomics often involve comparative analyses—differences between two or more genotypes and two or more diets—the results from this field of research will have direct application for improving the health of the large numbers of people who lack adequate nutrition, as well as those who overconsume.

ACKNOWLEDGMENTS

This work was supported by the National Center for Minority Health and Health Disparities Center of Excellence in Nutritional Genomics Grant MD-00222 and NutraGenomics (Chicago, IL).

REFERENCES

1. BEJA-PEREIRA, A., G. LUIKART, P.R. ENGLAND, et al. 2003. Gene–culture coevolution between cattle milk protein genes and human lactase genes. Nat. Genet. **35:** 311–313.
2. BROCKMANN, G.A. & M.R. BEVOVA. 2002. Using mouse models to dissect the genetics of obesity. Trends Genet. **18:** 367–376.
3. BULUN, S.E., T.M. PRICE, J. AITKEN, et al. 1993. A link between breast cancer and local estrogen biosynthesis suggested by quantification of breast adipose tissue aromatase cytochrome P450 transcripts using competitive polymerase chain reaction after reverse transcription. J. Clin. Endocrinol. Metab. **77:** 1622–1628. [Published erratum. 1994.] J. Clin. Endocrinol. Metab. **78:**494.
4. CHAKRAVARTHY, M.V. & F.W. BOOTH. 2004. Eating, exercise, and "thrifty" genotypes: Connecting the dots toward an evolutionary understanding of modern chronic diseases. J. Appl. Physiol. **96:** 3–10.
5. CHAWLA, A., J.J. REPA, R.M. EVANS, et al. 2001. Nuclear receptors and lipid physiology: Opening the x-files. Science **294:** 1866–1870.

6. DAUNCEY, M.J., P. WHITE, K.A. BURTON *et al.* 2001. Nutrition–hormone receptor–gene interactions: implications for development and disease. Proc Nutr Soc. **60:** 63–72.

7. DONG, Z. 2000. Effects of food factors on signal transduction pathways. Biofactors **12:** 17–28.

8. EKINS, S., L. MIRNY, & E.G. SCHUETZ. 2002. A ligand-based approach to understanding selectivity of nuclear hormone receptors pxr, car, fxr, lxralpha, and lxrbeta. Pharm. Res. **19:** 1788–1800.

9. ENATTAH, N.S., T. SAHI, E. TERWILLIGER, *et al.* 2002. Identification of a variant associated with adult-type hypolactasia. Nat. Genet. **30:** 233–237.

10. FERGUSON, L.R. & J. KAPUT. 2004. Nutrigenomics and the New Zealand food industry. Food New Zealand [journal of the New Zealand Institute of Food Science and Technology]: 29–36.

11. FLINT, J. & R. MOTT. 2001. Finding the molecular basis of quantitative traits: Successes and pitfalls. Nat. Rev. Genet. **2:** 437–445.

12. FLOREZ, J.C., J. HIRSCHHORN & D. ALTSHULER. 2003. The inherited basis of diabetes mellitus: implications for the genetic analysis of complex traits. Annu. Rev. Genomics Hum. Genet. **4:** 257–291.

13. FOGG-JOHNSON, N. & J. KAPUT. 2003. Nutrigenomics: An emerging scientific discipline. Food Technol. **57:** 61–67.

14. FRANCIS, G.A., E. FAYARD, F. PICARD, *et al.* 2003. Nuclear receptors and the control of metabolism. Annu. Rev. Physiol. **65:** 261–311.

15. GHOSH, S., S.M. PALMER, N.R. RODRIGUES, *et al.* 1993. Polygenic control of autommimune diabetes in nonobese diabetes. Nature Genet. **3:** 404–409.

16. GUTENDORF, B. & J. WESTENDORF. 2001. Comparison of an array of in vitro assays for the assessment of the estrogenic potential of natural and synthetic estrogens, phytoestrogens and xenoestrogens. Toxicology **166:** 79–89.

17. ITOH, Y., Y. KAWAMATA, M. HARADA, *et al.* 2003. Free fatty acids regulate insulin secretion from pancreatic beta cells through gpr40. Nature **422:** 173–176.

18. JACOBS, M.N. & D.F. LEWIS. 2002. Steroid hormone receptors and dietary ligands: A selected review. Proc. Nutr. Soc. **61:** 105–122.

19. KAGAWA, Y., Y. YANAGISAWA, K. HASEGAWA, *et al.* 2002. Single nucleotide polymorphisms of thrifty genes for energy metabolism: Evolutionary origins and prospects for intervention to prevent obesity-related diseases. Biochem. Biophys. Res. Commun. **295:** 207–222.

20. KAPUT, J. 2004. Diet–disease gene interactions. Nutrition **20** (Nutrigenomics): 26–31.

21. KAPUT, J. & R. RODRIGUEZ. 2004. Nutritional genomics: The next frontier in the post-genomic era. Physiological Genomics **16:** 166–177.

22. KAPUT, J., D. SWARTZ, E. PAISLEY, *et al.* 1994. Diet–disease interactions at the molecular level: an experimental paradigm. J. Nutr. **124:** 1296S–1305S.

23. KUIPER, G.G., B. CARLSSON, K. GRANDIEN, *et al.* 1997. Comparison of the ligand binding specificity and transcript tissue distribution of estrogen receptors alpha and beta. Endocrinology **138:** 863–870.

24. LIEBERMAN, L.S. 2003. Dietary, evolutionary, and modernizing influences on the prevalence of type 2 diabetes. Annu. Rev. Nutr. **23:** 345-377.

25. LINDER, C.C. 2001. The influence of genetic background on spontaneous and genetically engineered mouse models of complex diseases. Lab. Anim. (NY) **30:** 34–39.

26. MOORE, L.B., B. GOODWIN, S.A. JONES, *et al.* 2000. St. John's wort induces hepatic drug metabolism through activation of the pregnane X receptor. Proc. Natl. Acad. Sci. USA. **97:** 7500–7502.
27. PAGEL, M. & R. MACE. 2004. The cultural wealth of nations. Nature **428:** 275–278.
28. PAISLEY, E.A., E. I. PARK, D.A. SWARTZ, *et al.* 1996. Temporal-regulation of serum lipids and stearoyl CoA desaturase and lipoprotein lipase mRNA in BALB/cHnn mice. J. Nutr. **126:** 2730–2737.
29. PARK, E.I., E.A. PAISLEY, H.J. MANGIAN *et al.* 1997. Lipid level and type alter stearoyl CoA desaturase mRNA abundance differently in mice with distinct susceptibilities to diet-influenced diseases. J. Nutr. **127:** 566–573.
30. PENNACCHIO, L.A. 2003. Insights from human/mouse genome comparisons. Mamm. Genome **14:** 429–436.
31. PIANETTI, S., S. GUO, K.T. KAVANAGH, *et al.* 2002. Green tea polyphenol epigallocatechin-3 gallate inhibits her-2/neu signaling, proliferation, and transformed phenotype of breast cancer cells. Cancer Res. **62:** 652–655.
32. RISCH, N., S. GHOSH, & J.A. TODD. 1993. Statistical evaluation of multiple-locus linkage data in experimental species and its relevance to human studies: application to nonobese diabetic (nod) mouse and human insulin-dependent diabetes mellitus (iddm). Am. J. Hum. Genet. **53:** 702–714.
33. SONG, Y.S., C. JIN & E.H. PARK. 2000. Identification of metabolites of phytosterols in rat feces using gc/ms. Arch. Pharm. Res. **23:** 599–604.
34. SWARTZ, D.A., E.I. PARK, W.J. VISEK *et al.* 1996. The e subunit gene of murine f1f0-ATP synthase. Genomic sequence, chromosomal mapping, and diet regulation. J. Biol. Chem. **271:** 20942–20948.
35. TISHKOFF, S.A. & S.M. WILLIAMS. 2002. Genetic analysis of African populations: Human evolution and complex disease. Nat. Rev. Genet. **3:** 611–621.
36. VOISEY, J. & A. VAN DAAL. 2002. Agouti: from mouse to man, from skin to fat. Pigment Cell Res. **15:** 10–18.
37. WANG, Y., C.B. HARVEY, W.S. PRATt *et al.* 1995. The lactase persistence/nonpersistence polymorphism is controlled by a cis-acting element. Hum. Mol. Genet. **4:** 657–662.
38. WENTWORTH, J.M., M. AGOSTINI, J. LOVE, *et al.* 2000. St John's wort, a herbal antidepressant, activates the steroid X receptor. J. Endocrinol. **166:** R11–R16.
39. WILLETT, W. 2002. Isocaloric diets are of primary interest in experimental and epidemiological studies. Int. J. Epidemiol. **31:** 694–695.
40. WILLETT, W.C. 2002. Balancing life-style and genomics research for disease prevention. Science **296:** 695–698.
41. WOLFF, G.L., R.L. KODELL, J.A. KAPUT *et al.* 1999. Caloric restriction abolishes enhanced metabolic efficiency induced by ectopic agouti protein in yellow mice. Proc. Soc. Exp. Biol. Med. **221:** 99–104.
42. WOLFF, G.L., D.W. ROBERTS & K.G. MOUNTJOY. 1999. Physiological consequences of ectopic agouti gene expression: the yellow obese mouse syndrome. Physiol. Genomics **1:** 151–163.
43. KAPUT, J., K.G. KLEIN, E.J. REYES, *et al.* 2004. Identification of genes contributing to the obese yellow A^{vy} phenotype: caloric restriction, genotype, diet X genotype interactions. Physiological Genomics **18:** 316–324.

Effects of Testosterone on Cognitive and Brain Aging in Elderly Men

SCOTT D. MOFFAT

Institute of Gerontology and Department of Psychology, Wayne State University, Detroit, Michigan, USA

ABSTRACT: Older age is associated with functional declines throughout the body, including some aspects of cognitive performance. While dementia develops in only some elderly individuals, declines in cognitive functioning have an impact on daily living for many others. There are individual differences in age-related cognitive changes, however, and the factors that contribute to this variability have not been well-characterized. Recent evidence suggesting that age-related alterations in the endocrine environment may modulate cognitive changes has generated considerable interest. Currently, there is a discordance between the rapidly expanding number of studies of the possible neuroprotective effects of estrogens in postmenopausal women, and the relative dearth of analogous research on the putative effects of testosterone on cognitive and brain function in older men. This paper reviews the extant literature and reports new findings on the effects of testosterone loss and supplementation on cognitive and brain function in elderly men. Preliminary evidence suggests that testosterone loss may be a risk factor for cognitive decline and possibly for dementia. Conversely, the maintenance of higher testosterone levels either endogenously or through exogenous supplementation may prove beneficial for cognitive and brain function in elderly men. However, most studies are associational in nature and the intervention studies are of short-duration testosterone exposure in small samples of subjects. Large-scale placebo-controlled intervention studies are required to resolve ambiguities in the literature. Testosterone intervention to ameliorate cognitive decline may be warranted only when the efficacy and safety of longer-term use is firmly established.

KEYWORDS: testosterone; androgen; Alzheimer's disease; dementia; memory; aging; hippocampus

Older age is associated with functional declines throughout the body, including some aspects of cognitive performance. However, there are marked individual differences in age-related cognitive changes, and the factors that

Addresss for correspondence: Scott D. Moffat, Ph.D., Institute of Gerontology, 87 East Ferry Street, Detroit 48202, MI. Voice: 313-577-2297; fax: 313-875-0127.
moffat@wayne.edu

Ann. N.Y. Acad. Sci. 1055: 80–92 (2005). © 2005 New York Academy of Sciences.
doi: 10.1196/annals.1323.014

contribute to this variability have not been well-characterized. Recent evidence suggests that the hormonal environment may modulate these age-related cognitive changes. For example, there is some evidence that post-menopausal hormone replacement therapy (HRT) may exert beneficial effects on specific cognitive functions, but this remains controversial. In men, testosterone (T) levels decline precipitously between the ages of 30 and 80; results from both epidemiologic research and T replacement studies suggest that this progressive decline in testosterone secretion in aging men contributes to selective losses in memory and cognitive function. In order to fully understand the neurocognitive effects of steroid hormones, it is imperative that the cognitive and neural effects of testosterone loss and its subsequent replacement be fully characterized. Evidence for the possible neurotrophic and neuroprotective effects of testosterone come from investigations in humans and in non-human species.

EFFECTS OF TESTOSTERONE ON BEHAVIORAL AND NEURAL SYSTEMS

In non-human species, a number of behavioral systems are responsive to gonadal steroids in both adult and developing animals. Among the diverse behavioral systems whose development and expression are sensitive to gonadal steroids include sexual and maternal behavior, overall activity levels, open field activity, aggression, juvenile play, feeding and taste preferences, motor behavior, and song production in songbirds.[1-3] An important element in understanding the effects of testosterone on the nervous system is that many of its behavioral and anatomical effects occur after it has been converted to its metabolically active derivatives, estradiol (E) or dihydrotestosterone (DHT) by means of the enzymes aromatase and 5-α reductase, respectively. Thus, testosterone may interact not only with androgen receptors, but also with E receptors, and hence, its administration may in some circumstances parallel the effects of E throughout the nervous system.

Of particular interest to researchers investigating hormonal contributions to human abilities is the observation that regions of the rat brain thought to subserve aspects of spatial learning and memory, including the hippocampus, have been shown to be affected by gonadal hormones. The hippocampus contains high concentrations of androgen receptors[4] and administration of testosterone to females during critical periods of development enhances spatial learning while castration in males impairs maze learning.[5-8]

Testosterone exerts an early organizational effect on the development of the hypothalamus,[9] the cerebral cortex,[10] the hippocampus,[5] and other cerebral structures, and several observations suggest that testosterone is also capable of modulating neural systems in adult animals. For example, testosterone loss in aging mice is associated with spatial learning deficits, which are reversed by administration of testosterone.[11] Moreover, the physiological effects of testosterone strongly suggest that it may serve as an important neuroprotective and neurotrophic factor. These properties of testosterone make it a possible candidate for the prevention and/or amelioration of cognitive decline. For example, androgen treatment prevents N-methyl-D-aspartate (NMDA) excitotoxicity in hippocampal neurons[12] and may facilitate recovery after injury by promoting fiber outgrowth and sprouting.[13] Administration of testosterone increases nerve growth factor (NGF) levels in the hippocampus, and induces an upregulation of NGF receptors in the forebrain. [14] Testosterone may also have important inhibitory effects on the expression of amyloid, one of the principal neuropathologic hallmarks of Alzheimer's disease (AD). Testosterone decreases amyloid secretion from rat cortical neurons[15] and reduces amyloid-induced neurotoxicity in cultured hippocampal neurons.[16]

Although work investigating the *neurophysiological* effects of testosterone in humans is in its infancy, preliminary work supports the findings from the animal literature. In humans, suppression of testosterone for treatment of prostate cancer resulted in a two-fold *increase* in plasma amyloid concentrations in elderly men, suggesting that higher levels of endogenous testosterone may reduce plasma amyloid concentrations in humans.[17] In another important study, Hammond *et al.*[18] found that testosterone was protective of human primary neurons in culture, providing the most direct evidence for neuroprotective effects of testosterone on human neural tissue.

Taken together, these findings suggest that testosterone may exert important neurotrophic and neuroprotective effects, making it a potential therapeutic agent for the treatment of cognitive decline in elderly men. Additionally, studies in non-human species compellingly demonstrate that testosterone affects various aspects of behavior including learning and memory. It is, therefore, reasonable to investigate whether such effects may be present in humans as well.

EFFECTS OF TESTOSTERONE ON HUMAN COGNITIVE FUNCTION

The large and expanding literature investigating the effects of hormone replacement therapy in women contrasts sharply to the state of science of the endocrinology of men's aging. There is a comparative dearth of research elucidating the effects of testosterone on cognitive and neural function. However, as with the research undertaken in non-human species, there is evidence that testosterone may have important behavioral and cognitive effects in humans. Among younger adults, the effects of testosterone on visuo-spatial performance has been suggested by enhanced performance in females exposed prenatally to excess androgens[19,20] and reduced spatial performance in young males with hypogonadism.[21] The majority of investigations examining the association between testosterone levels and cognition have been studies in young adult men and women. Our own data[22] indicated that females with higher testosterone levels outperform those with lower levels of testosterone, while the reverse may be true in young males. Results from other[23-25] but not all [6,27] studies have reported a similar inverted U-shaped relationship between testosterone and spatial cognition in samples of young adults. Language-related measures such as verbal fluency show no significant relationship to testosterone. These correlational studies in young adults relating naturally occurring individual differences in testosterone to cognitive abilities reliably implicate spatial cognition as the domain of cognitive function most sensitive to testosterone concentrations.

Several studies have now examined the association between testosterone and cognition in older men. The progressive decline in testosterone levels with age[28,29] raises the question of whether hypoandrogenism is associated with age-related declines in cognitive functions. Morley *et al.* assessed androgen levels and cognitive performance in a sample of 56 men aged 21–84 years and found that age-related decreases in bioavailable testosterone predicted age-related decline in visual and verbal memory.[30] This study is one of the few studies to report *longitudinal* findings relating testosterone to rates of cognitive decline. Longitudinal designs are particularly important in this field as this is the only way to acquire data on within-individual *rates of change* in cognitive function, which may be a very important factor for assessing who may be a greatest risk for later acquisition of AD. In one epidemiologic study of 547 men age 59–89 years,[31] higher bioavailable testosterone concentrations were found in men who scored better on a measure of long-term verbal memory. In a second study, the relationship between endogenous steroid levels and cognitive performance was investigated in 383 women, aged 55 to 89 years.[32] Women with higher scores on mental status had significantly higher total and bioavailable testosterone levels.

In a series of comprehensive studies from the Baltimore Longitudinal Study of Aging (BLSA), we have investigated the cognitive and neural consequences of testosterone loss in aging men. In the first study,[33] we investigated age-associated decreases in endogenous testosterone concentrations and declines in neuro-psychological performance among 407 men aged 50 to 91 years. The men in the study were followed *longitudinally* for an average of 10 years, with assessments of multiple cognitive domains and contemporaneous determination of total serum testosterone, sex hormone–binding globulin (SHBG), and a calculated free testosterone index. In this study, higher free testosterone was associated with higher scores on visual and verbal memory and visuospatial functioning and with a reduced rate of decline in visual memory. No relations were observed between testosterone and measures of verbal knowledge, general mental status, or depressive symptoms.

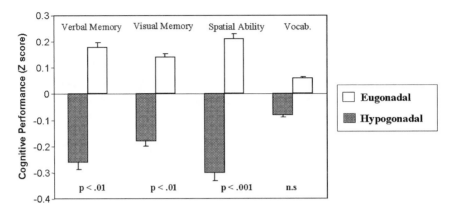

FIGURE 1. Cognitive performance in hypogondal and eugonadal men in four domains of cognitive performance. All cognitive test results are presented in standard scores. After age and other relevant factors (see text) were controlled, hypogonadal men performed more poorly than eugonadal men on measures of verbal and visual memory and spatial cognition.

In a second component of the same study, we classified men as either hypogonadal (less than the 2.5 percentile of men under 40), or eugonadal based on established guidelines.[29] Comparison of the two groups of men revealed higher spatial cognition, verbal memory, and visual memory function among the eugonadal men (FIG. 1). In addition, in longitudinal analyses, we observed a reduced rate of decline in visual memory among eugonadal men (FIG. 2). The effect sizes from these comparisons were substantial. For example, the difference between hypogonadal and eugonadal men on spatial cognition was one-half of a standard deviation (d = 0.52). These results demonstrate a possible beneficial effect of high circulating free testosterone concentrations in older men on specific domains of cognitive performance and cognitive decline. Although these data cannot confirm a causal impact of testosterone on neuropsychological outcome, we took every measure to control health-related factors that may potentially affect testosterone concentrations or cognitive performance, including smoking, alcohol use, body mass index, heart disease and diabetes status, age, and education levels. Moreover, individuals with cancer, dementia, or other neurologic or psychiatric problems were excluded from the study. Nevertheless, because of the associational nature of our and other studies, we cannot eliminate the possibility that low T/free T levels may serve as a marker for, rather than a causative factor in, age-related cognitive decline.

In a neuroimaging study of a subsample of these same men from the Baltimore Longitudinal Study of Aging, we quantified long-term testosterone con-

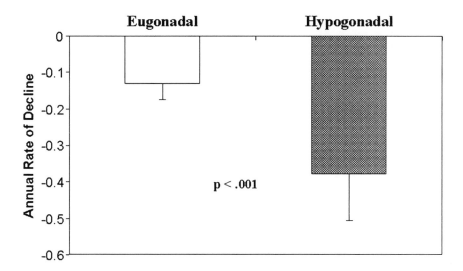

FIGURE 2. Annual rate of decline in visual memory as a function of hypogonadal or eugonadal status. Men classified as hypogonadal had a steeper rate of decline in visual memory than did eugonadal men.

centration in association with regional cerebral blood flow (rCBF) as determined by positron emission tomography (PET). We found that men with higher endogenous free T had increased blood flow in the hippocampus bilaterally. This study converges with our cognitive findings in the full BLSA sample in demonstrating that high levels of endogenous free testosterone is associated with improved memory and spatial cognition and increased resting activation of the hippocampus. This is significant as the hippocampus plays a critical role in memory and possibly in spatial cognitive processing. The latter neuroimaging study may provide the beginnings of physiological explanation for the possible beneficial effects of free testosterone on cognitive function.

A related question concerning cognitive aging is whether age-related testosterone decline may be a risk factor for the development and diagnosis of Alzheimer's disease (AD). Some recent cross-sectional studies have reported lower testosterone concentrations in men diagnosed with AD.[34–37] A problem with studies assessing androgen levels in individuals who have already been diagnosed with AD is that the depleted testosterone levels could be a consequence rather than a cause of the disease. For example, degnerative brain changes in AD could potentially alter hypothalamic-pituitary-gonadal axis function and result in altered steroid hormone levels. Thus, it is important to evaluate hormone levels *prior* to the diagnosis of AD to be more certain that lower androgen levels do not follow CNS changes in Alzheimer's disease.

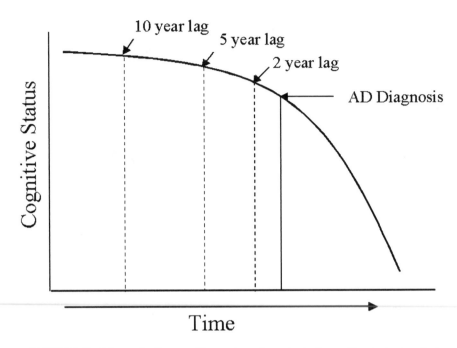

FIGURE 3. Schematic diagram illustrating a hypothetical cognitive trajectory in individuals who are ultimately diagnosed with Alzheimer's disease. In our study assessing testosterone levels in AD, we restricted our testosterone assays only to those serum samples that were collected *before* the date of AD diagnosis. We performed three analyses, restricting assays to those samples that were collected 2, 5 or 10 years prior to diagnosis. This was done to minimize the possibility that reduced testosterone levels in AD may be a consequence rather than a cause of the disease.

The most convincing study to date suggesting that testosterone could protect against AD and cognitive decline was part of the Baltimore Longitudinal Study of Aging. Importantly, in this prospective longitudinal study, we quantified long-term testosterone concentrations in individuals prior to the diagnosis of dementia.[38] This was done by restricting assays only to those blood samples that were provided 2, 5 and 10 years prior to the diagnosis of AD diagnosis (FIG. 3). Consistent with the results of other studies, we observed lower free testosterone levels in individuals diagnosed with AD compared to controls (FIG 4). More specifically, the results of this study revealed an approximately 10% reduction in the risk for AD for each unit increase in free testosterone. These results were robust with respect to restricting testosterone values to 2, 5 and 10 years prior to AD diagnosis. The restriction of testosterone observations to as long as 10 years *prior* to diagnosis of AD makes it very unlikely that the reduced testosterone concentrations observed in persons with Alzheimer's disease was a result of AD pathology. This study pro-

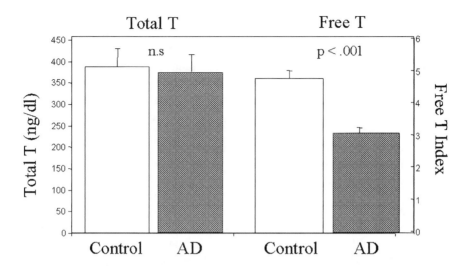

FIGURE 4. Mean total testosterone (T) and mean free T levels in individuals diagnosed with AD and non-demented controls. There was no difference between AD patients and controls in total T, but we observed significantly lower free T levels in patients with AD than in controls. There was an approximately 10% reduced risk for AD for each unit increase in free T.

vides the clearest evidence to date that altered testosterone levels in AD may precede rather than follow diagnosis. Indeed it suggests that lower testosterone levels may be evident quite early in those individuals who go on to develop dementia years later. Care was taken to control for health-related factors that may potentially affect testosterone concentrations or cognitive performance. Nevertheless, because of the associational nature of observational studies, the possibility that low T/free T levels may serve as a co-morbid side-effect of dementia, rather than a specific causative factor, cannot be eliminated.

An interesting possibility is that relations between testosterone and cognitive function and dementia could be mediated in part by age-related alterations in levels of gonadotropins. In response to lower testosterone with age in men, the pituitary gland may increase secretion of luteinizing hormone (LH) and follicle-stimulating hormone (FSH) to increase androgen levels.[28] One hypothesis argues that high levels of gonadotropins may have direct and deleterious effects on brain function.[39] Levels of gonadotropins were found to be increased in men with AD compared with age-matched controls.[40] These authors further reported a significant increase in LH in pyramidal neurons and neurofibrillary tangles of AD brains compared to age-matched control brains.[40] These data could be interpreted to suggest that high levels of gonadotropins, rather than low levels of testosterone *per se*, may be implicated in pathological aging processes. Of course, hypotheses regarding the role of testosterone and gonadotropins in human aging need not be mutually exclusive. Low levels of testosterone may prove to be a risk factor for brain health by virtue of depriving the brain of an important neuroprotective agent, and high levels of gonadotropins could represent a concomitant risk factor. This research is still in the preliminary stages and future studies may be able to determine relative contributions of androgens and gonadotropins to cognitive and brain aging.

To overcome the drawbacks that are inherent in associational studies, it is essential to perform randomized intervention studies to more conclusively investigate the possible cognitive effects of testosterone. A few studies have adopted such an approach in evaluating this issue. In a double-blind placebo-controlled study,[41] cognitive performance was investigated in a community sample of older men to whom testosterone was administered via scrotal patch (15 mg/day) for 3 months to treat androgen deficiency. Men who received testosterone had selectively enhanced Block Design scores compared to men receiving a placebo, demonstrating that testosterone may improve spatial-constructional abilities in elderly men. In a more recent placebo-controlled trial,[42] 150 mg of testosterone enanthate or placebo was administered once per week by intramuscular injection to a sample of older men averaging 67 years of age. These investigators found that men who received testosterone supplementation showed a reduction in working memory errors compared to placebo-treated men. In a recent testosterone intervention study conducted in elderly men, Cherrier et al. found improved verbal memory, improved spatial ability, and improved route recall in men who received 6 weeks of testosterone enanthate (100 mg/week, intramuscular injection).[43] In a recent study examining the efficacy of testosterone intervention in men with AD and mild cognitive impairment (a possible prodromal phase of AD), men were administered 100 mg per week of testosterone enanthate by weekly injection for 13 weeks.[44] Men in the study showed selective enhancement of spatial memory, constructional skills, and verbal memory. This may be the first study to demonstrate some enhancement of cognitive function in AD by androgen intervention therapy.

However, not all studies of testosterone intervention have reported improvements in cognition. One such study[45] found that one year of testosterone supplementation did not improve memory or verbal fluency scores. Whether a battery that included more sensitive measures of spatial memory and spatial cognition may have resulted in positive findings could not be evaluated in this study. A second study[46] found no effect of a single injection of testosterone on cognitive testing one week later. This single testosterone injection and 1-week duration of exposure may have been insufficient to detect cognitive effects.

The results of observational studies, taken together with recent small-scale testosterone intervention trials in elderly men, suggest that the progressive

physiological decline in testosterone secretion with aging contributes to selective losses in cognitive function. Preliminary data from well-designed placebo-controlled testosterone intervention studies suggests that these deficits
may be reversed, at least in part, by short-term testosterone supplementation.
However, we are far from concluding unequivocally that testosterone may enhance brain and cognitive function. The reasons for this are two-fold. First,
epidemiologic studies suffer from lack of control of some extraneous variables that are inherent in all studies of this design, and controlling for these
factors after the fact in advanced statistical models does not substitute for random assignment. Even when considering the extant placebo-controlled trials,
present findings that are less than conclusive. The studies provide important
converging data but they tend to based on small samples of men and investigate testosterone interventions that are relatively short in duration. Moreover,
because of their short duration and limited scope, they have not adequately
evaluated the safety of testosterone intervention on other body systems. What
is needed in this field are large, well-controlled intervention studies assessing
the effects of testosterone on multiple body systems. Indeed, the Institute of
Medicine (IOM) of the National Academy of Sciences recently recommended that clinical trials be conducted in men 65 years of age and over with testosterone concentrations below the physiologic levels of young adult men.
This report specifically identified cognitive function as one of four target areas in need of clinical investigation. Currently there is some cause for opti-
mism that testosterone may aid the treatment of cognitive and neural
dysfunction in some aging men. However it would be premature to advocate
testosterone intervention to prevent or ameliorate cognitive decline unless
and until research clearly bears out both the efficacy and safety of so doing.

REFERENCES

1. BEATTY, W.W. 1992. Gonadal hormones and sex differences in nonreproduc-
   tive behaviors. *In* Handbook of Behavioral Neurology Volume II: Sexual Differentiation. A.A. Gerall, H. Moltz & I.L. Ward IL, Eds.: 85–128. Plenum
   Press. New York.
2. BECKER, J.B., S.M. BREEDLOVE & D. CREWS. 1992. Behavioral Endocrinology.
   MIT Press. Cambridge, MA.
3. GOY, R.W. & B.S. MCEWEN. 1980. Sexual Differentiation of the Brain. MIT
   Press. Cambridge, MA.
4. KERR, J.E., R.J. ALLORE, S.G. BECK & R.J. HANDA. 1995. Distribution and
   hormonal regulation of androgen receptor (AR) and AR messenger ribonu-
   cleic acid in the rat hippocampus. Endocrinology **136:** 3213–3221.
5. ROOF, R.L. & M.D. HAVENS. 1992. Testosterone improves maze performance
   and induces development of a male hippocampus in females. Brain Res. **572:**
   310–313.

6. STEWART, J., A. SKVARENINA & J. POTTIER. 1975. Effects of neonatal androgens on open-field behavior and maze learning in the prepubescent and adult rat. Physiol. Behav. **14:** 291–295.
7. WILLIAMS, C.L. & W.H. MECK. 1991. The organizational effects of gonadal steroids on sexually dimorphic spatial ability. Psychoneuroendocrinology **16:** 155–176.
8. WILLIAMS, C.L., A.M. BARNETT & W.H. MECK. 1990. Organizational effects of early gonadal secretions on sexual differentiation in spatial memory. Behav. Neurosci. **104:** 84–97.
9. JACOBSON, C.D., V.J. CSERNUS, J.E. SHRYNE & R.A. GORSKI. 1981. The influence of gonadectomy, androgen exposure, or a gonadal graft in the neonatal rat on the volume of the sexually dimorphic nucleus of the preoptic area. J. Neurosci. **1:** 1142–1147.
10. DIAMOND, M.C. 1991. Hormonal effects on the development or cerebral lateralization. Psychoneuroendocrinology **16:** 121–129.
11. FLOOD, J.F., S.A. FARR, F.E. KAISER, *et al.* 1995. Age-related decrease of plasma testosterone in SAMP8 mice: replacement improves age-related impairment of learning and memory. Physiol Behav. **57:** 669–673.
12. POULIOT, W.A., R.J. HANDA & S.G. BECK. 1996. Androgen modulates N-methyl-D-aspartate-mediated depolarization in CA1 hippocampal pyramidal cells. Synapse **23:** 10–19.
13. MORSE, J.K., S.T. DEKOSKY & S.W. SCHEFF. 1992. Neurotrophic effects of steroids on lesion-induced growth in the hippocampus. II. Hormone replacement. Exp. Neurol. **118:** 47–52.
14. TIRASSA, P., I. THIBLIN, G. AGREN, *et al.* 1997. High-dose anabolic androgenic steroids modulate concentrations of nerve growth factor and expression of its low affinity receptor (p75-NGFr) in male rat brain. J. Neurosci. Res. **47:** 198–207.
15. GOURAS, G.K., H. XU, R.S. GROSS, *et al.* 2000. Testosterone reduces neuronal secretion of Alzheimer's beta-amyloid peptides. Proc. Natl. Acad. Sci. USA **97:** 1202–1205.
16. PIKE, C.J. 2001. Testosterone attenuates beta-amyloid toxicity in cultured hippocampal neurons. Brain Res. **919:** 160–165.
17. GANDY, S., O.P. ALMEIDA, J. FONTE, *et al.* 2001. Chemical andropause and amyloid-beta peptide. JAMA **285:** 2195–2196.
18. HAMMOND, J., Q. LE, C. GOODYER, *et al.* 2001. Testosterone-mediated neuroprotection through the androgen receptor in human primary neurons. J. Neurochem. **77:** 1319–1326.
19. RESNICK, S.M., S.A. BERENBAUM, I.I. GOTTESMAN & T.J. BOUCHARD. 1986. Early hormonal influences on cognitive functioning in congenital adrenal hyperplasia. Dev. Psychol. **22:** 191–198.
20. HAMPSON, E., J.F. ROVET & D. ALTMANN. 1998. Spatial reasoning in children with congenital adrenal hyperplasia due to 21-hydroxylase deficiency. Developmental Neuropsychology **14:** 299–320.
21. HIER, D. & W. CROWLEY. 1982. Spatial abilities in androgen deficient men. N. Engl. J. Med. **302:** 1202–1205.
22. MOFFAT, S.D. & E. HAMPSON. 1996. A curvilinear relationship between testosterone and spatial cognition in humans: possible influence of hand preference. Psychoneuroendocrinology **21:** 323–337.

23. SHUTE, V.J., J.W. PELLEGRINO, L. HUBERT & R.W. REYNOLDS. 1983. The relationship between androgen levels and human spatial ability. Bull. Psychonom. Soc. **21:** 465–468.
24. GOUCHIE, C. & D. KIMURA. 1991. The relationship between testosterone levels and cognitive ability patterns. Psychoneuroendocrinology **16:** 323–334.
25. NEAVE, N., M. MENAGED & D.R. WEIGHTMAN. 1999. Sex differences in cognition: the role of testosterone and sexual orientation. Brain Cogn. **41:** 245–262.
26. CHRISTIANSEN, K. & R. KNUSSMANN. 1987. Sex hormones and cognitive functioning in men. Neuropsychobiology **18:** 27–36.
27. SILVERMAN, I., D. KASTUK, J. CHOI & K. PHILLIPS. 1999. Testosterone levels and spatial ability in men. Psychoneuroendocrinology **24:** 813–822.
28. LAMBERTS, S.W., A.W. VAN DEN BELD & A.J. VAN DER LELY 1997. The endocrinology of aging. Science **278:** 419–424.
29. HARMAN, S.M., E.J. METTER, J.D. TOBIN, et al. 2001. Longitudinal effects of aging on serum total and free testosterone levels in healthy men. Baltimore Longitudinal Study of Aging. J. Clin. Endocrinol. Metab. **86:** 724–731.
30. MORLEY, J.E., F. KAISER, W.J. RAUM, et al. 1997. Potentially predictive and manipulable blood serum correlates of aging in the healthy human male: progressive decreases in bioavailable testosterone, dehydroepiandrosterone sulfate, and the ratio of insulin-like growth factor 1 to growth hormone. Proc. Natl. Acad. Sci. USA **94:** 7537–7542.
31. BARRETT-CONNOR, E., D. GOODMAN-GRUEN & B. PATAY. 1999. Endogenous sex hormones and cognitive function in older men. J. Clin. Endocrinol. Metab. **84:** 3681–3685.
32. BARRETT-CONNOR, E. & D. GOODMAN-GRUEN. 1999. Cognitive function and endogenous sex hormones in older women. J. Am. Geriatr. Soc. **47:** 1289–1293.
33. MOFFAT, S.D., A.B. ZONDERMAN, E.J. METTER, et al. 2002. Longitudinal assessment of serum free testosterone concentration predicts memory performance and cognitive status in elderly men. J. Clin. Endocrinol. Metab. **87:** 5001–5007.
34. HOGERVORST, E., J. WILLIAM, M. BUDGE, et al. 2001. Serum total testosterone is lower in men with Alzheimer's disease. Neuroendocrinol. Lett. **22:** 163–168.
35. HOGERVORST, E., S. BANDELOW, M. COMBRINCK & A.D. SMITH. 2004. Low free testosterone is an independent risk factor for Alzheimer's disease. Exp. Gerontol. **39:** 1633–1639.
36. PAOLETTI, A.M., S. CONGIA. S. LELLO, et al. 2004. Low androgenization index in elderly women and elderly men with Alzheimer's disease. Neurology **62:** 301–303.
37. WATANABE, T., S. KOBA, M. KAWAMURA, et al. 2004. Small dense low-density lipoprotein and carotid atherosclerosis in relation to vascular dementia. Metabolism **53:** 476–482.
38. MOFFAT, S.D., A.B. ZONDERMAN, E.J. METTER, et al. 2004. Free testosterone and risk for Alzheimer disease in older men. Neurology **62:** 188–193.
39. MEETHAL, S.V., M.A. SMITH, R.L. BOWEN & C.S. ATWOOD. 2005. The gonadotropin connection in Alzheimer's disease. Endocrine **26:** 317–326.
40. BOWEN, R.L., M.A. SMITH, P.L. HARRIS, et al. 2002. Elevated luteinizing hormone expression colocalizes with neurons vulnerable to Alzheimer's disease pathology. J. Neurosci. Res. **70:** 514–518.

41. JANOWSKY, J.S, S.K. OVIATT & E.S. ORWOLL. 1994. Testosterone influences spatial cognition in older men. Behav. Neurosci. **108:** 325–332.
42. JANOWSKY, J.S., B. CHAVEZ & E. ORWOLL. 2000. Sex steroids modify working memory. J. Cogn. Neurosci. **12:** 407–414.
43. CHERRIER, M.M., S. ASTHANA, S. PLYMATE, *et al.* 2001. Testosterone supplementation improves spatial and verbal memory in healthy older men. Neurology. **57:** 80–88.
44. CHERRIER, M.M., A.M. MATSUMOTO, J.K. AMORY, *et al.* 2005. Testosterone improves spatial memory in men with Alzheimer disease and mild cognitive impairment. Neurology **64:** 2063–2068.
45. SIH, R., J.E. MORLEY, F.E. KAISER, *et al.* 1997. Testosterone replacement in older hypogonadal men: a 12–month randomized controlled trial. J. Clin. Endocrinol. Metab. **82:** 1661–1667.
46. WOLF, O.T., R. PREUT, D.H. HELLHAMMER, *et al.* 2000. Testosterone and cognition in elderly men: a single testosterone injection blocks the practice effect in verbal fluency, but has no effect on spatial or verbal memory. Biol. Psychiatry **47:** 650–654.

Oxidative Stress Profiling

Part I. Its Potential Importance in the Optimization of Human Health

RICHARD G. CUTLER

Kronos Science Laboratories, Inc., Phoenix, Arizona 85016, USA

ABSTRACT: Steadily accumulating scientific evidence supports the general importance of oxidative damage of tissue and cellular components as a primary or secondary causative factor in many different human diseases and aging processes. Our goal has been to develop sensitive and reliable means to measure the oxidative damage and defense/repair status of an individual that could be easily used by a physician to determine whether there is an immediate or long-term increased health risk to their patients with regard to oxidative damage. We also sought to try to determine how this risk can best be reduced, and whether the prescribed therapy is working and how it might be best adjusted to optimize benefits. We have found that combining both an oxidative damage profile with a defense/repair profile produces the most reliable set of information to meet these objectives. Success is indicated by demonstrating the expected inverse correlation of oxidative stress vs. antioxidant status of a population of several hundred individuals. We also find support that oxidative stress status is under tight regulatory control for most individuals over a wide range of lifestyle variables including diet and exercise. Indeed only about 10% of the individuals analyzed appear to have unusually high oxidative stress levels. Only these individuals having the higher than normal levels of oxidative stress are the best responders to antioxidant supplements to lower their oxidative stress status to normal levels. We discuss the implications of these results for human application and review how current clinical studies are carried out to evaluate the benefits of antioxidant supplements in reducing the incidence of specific age-dependent disease.

KEYWORDS: oxidative stress; oxidative stress status; oxidative stress profiling; longevity-determinant genes; dysdifferentiation; evolution of longevity; aging; geriatrics

Address for correspondence: Richard G. Cutler, Longevity Sciences Group, Kronos Science Laboratories, Inc., 2222 E. Highland Avenue, Suite 220, Phoenix, AZ 85016. Voice: 602-778-7488; fax: 602-667-5623

richard.cutler@kronoslaboratory.com

Ann. N.Y. Acad. Sci. 1055: 93–135 (2005). © 2005 New York Academy of Sciences.
doi: 10.1196/annals.1323.027

OBJECTIVES

The aim of this paper is to look at:

- the general importance of oxidative damage to tissue and cellular components as a causative factor in different human diseases and aging processes; and the

- development of highly sensitive and reliable means to measure the oxidative damage and defense/repair status

INTRODUCTION

Much experimental data now exists in the scientific literature indicating the general importance of oxidative stress as a causative factor in many of the age-related human diseases as well as a causative factor for the aging process itself.[1–6] For example, risk factors for cardiovascular disease, many types of cancer, and diabetes are often also associated with the oxidative stress status of the individual.[7] Substantial correlative data also indicate a positive association of oxidative stress status with the aging rate of different species.[8–17] In model organisms used to study aging—such as yeast, nematode, *Drosophila* and mice—recent data have shown that increased resistance to oxidative stress gained as a result of simple genetic alterations can dramatically increase life span.[18–22]

The implications of these studies towards developing the means to optimize human health and longevity offer novel research and practical opportunities.[8,9,11,23–25] For example, it is well known all individuals do not live the same length of time. Many die in their 50s and 60s as a result of specific inherent weakness leading to diseases such as cancer, heart disease, or diabetes. Yet others are able to live healthy life spans up to age 80 years or more. Then there are the rare centenarian and supercentenarian individuals who are able to live healthy productive lives up to and well past 100 years of age.[26–43]

Why is this so? Could it be that the potential healthy life span of individuals is highly dependent on their life-long oxidative stress status, as appears to be the case across different species? To check out this possibility it would be useful to develop a noninvasive means to measure the oxidative stress status of an individual. A set of biochemical blood and urine assays could be developed to determine the oxidative stress profile, and we might see whether the information contained in such a profile could serve as useful markers of risk towards age-related disease or the potential for excellent health and longevity.

This oxidative stress profile would contain information providing a physician with the ability to determine whether the patient has an unusually high level of oxidative stress as well of indications of what could be done to lower it. On the basis of evidence indicating that each individual is unique with respect to genetics and lifestyle and therefore biology, effective and optimal lowering of an individual's oxidative stress status requires a broad set of analytical assays and a customized therapy program. This effort requires taking an individual through several repeated tests and trial therapies to arrive at the most effective therapy or dietary supplement schedule. One attractive aspect of this process is that the patient observes first hand whether the therapy or supplement recommend by the physician actually works and whether his or her oxidative stress status has been reduced or minimized.

At this time the long-term clinical studies necessary to prove that reduction of oxidative stress in humans will result in an increase their healthy life span have not been undertaken, but certainly we know of no *advantage* of oxidative damage nor any *disadvantage* of a low oxidative stress status. On the other hand, an extraordinary body of scientific evidence now indicates that unusually high levels of oxidative stress are associated with ill health, disease, and early death. Thus it is highly probable, if not proven, that some benefit would be realized. The more difficult question is the relation of lowering oxidative stress to an increase in general health status. Since the cost to lower oxidative stress is not likely to be high and there are essentially no toxic side effects, most individuals would likely choose to take the necessary steps to minimize their oxidative stress status. It could be viewed as a life insurance move with little to lose, but much potentially to gain.

The objective of this paper is to provide a brief background and update of our past work and experience to achieve this goal. First, I will briefly give an overview of human aging and longevity biology followed by evidence supporting the role of oxidative stress as a potentially important causative factor of aging. Secondly a brief review will follow of experiments used in developing the oxidative stress profile technique and its application at the Kronos Science Laboratory.

RECTANGULARIZATION OF THE HUMAN SURVIVAL CURVE

Much information can be gained about the nature of human aging processes by an examination of human survival over the past 10,000 years or so. A percent survival curve is where the percent survival of a given population of individuals is plotted as a function of the chronological age of a population.[26,27,44–47] Usually age starts at zero years (newborn individuals) and survival at 100%, and the curve moves downward with increasing chronological age until it reaches 0% survival at the age of death if the last member of the population. All causes of death are included in the calculation of the % survival fraction.

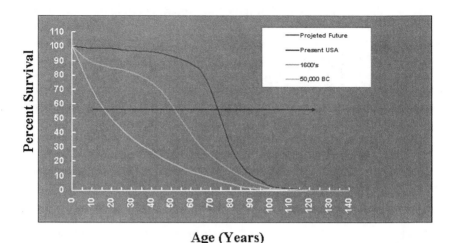

Age (Years)

FIGURE 1. Typical human survival curve.

The "mean survival" is where 50% of the original population has died and this has been defined as the "life expectancy" age of the population. When 0% survival is reached this is defined as the "maximum life span potential" (MLSP) or more recently the "life span" of the population. A typical human survival curve is shown in FIGURE 1.

For most of human history individuals rarely lived long enough to suffer from any decline in physiological activity due to the aging process.[48–51] This is common for all animals living in their natural ecological niche. Death is usually by predators or other external environmental hazards. So for most of human history, the survival curve is an exponentially declining one defined by the probability of death being a constant and independent of chronological age. Here the life expectancy (50% survival) of the human was about 25 years. Thus, at the age of 40 years, about 25% of the population is left and very few individuals ever reach ages past 60 years. So primitive populations of humans were essentially populations of youth, with very few individuals reaching the age where the aging process would begin to affect their general health status.

Rate of aging or life span is a species characteristic, whereas life expectancy is not. Therefore it must be the case that, over the past 50,000 years during which hominid populations were all *Homo sapiens,* that the innate aging rate of the human population was no different than it is today.[8–10] So the short life expectancy observed for these early human populations is largely a result of their high environmental hazards, not a faster aging rate. There is, however, always the possibility that a few individuals living under these primitive conditions would be simply lucky and reach a much greater age range, as we have today in developed countries, but this would be very rare.

However, as humans learned to decrease their environmental hazards by reducing deaths caused by predators, increasing quality of food on a year-round basis, and most importantly decreasing problems related to infectious disease, a steady increase in life expectancy occurred.[9] *But this increase occurred without an increase in life span.* As a result we observe an increasing rectangularization of the survival curve as we progress from the past to the present day. Interestingly, most of this rectangularization occurred recently, over the past 400 years.

This rectangularization of the survival curve, where life expectancy has steadily increased but maximum survival or life span has remained fixed, suggests that human survival is determined by two major factors. One is the intensity of the physical external environmental hazards and the other is the physiological endogenous aging rate of the human population. Thus today death occurring early in life up to an age of 60 to 70 years is largely due to random events related to environmental hazards or specific diseases that progress independently of the innate aging process. But as individuals steadily grow older chronologically, the rate of aging increases ever more rapidly, resulting in placing an upper maximum limit to life span for any human. This limit is about 120 years of age. Studies of human survival have therefore provided the first evidence of the existence of a physiological process common to all humans which has remained essentially unchanged and proceeds at the same rate over the history of mankind.

It is also important to note that most of the increase in human life expectancy has occurred over the past 400 years and that this increase has not resulted in a significant increase in healthy years of life span. This is because the aging process has always been proceeding at the same rate. So today, with a life expectancy of about 75 to 80 years, human populations are simply now living physiologically *older longer* and deeper into old age and not living physiologically *younger longer*, as is often believed. To live younger longer would require a decrease in the innate rate of the human aging processes and this has never occurred to our knowledge.

THE PHYSIOLOGY OF HUMAN AGING

Although survival curves are popular in measuring life span in human and model organisms, it is very important to realize that there is no information in a survival curve database that can provide insight as to what caused the death of the individuals in the population. That is, actuarial data of age at death contain no information concerning the cause of death. This rather simple and obvious fact has unfortunately been ignored by many investigators, who have mistakenly associated physiological aging rate with parameters defining the survival curve.[52,53]

The aging process and the rate of aging in mammalian species is best characterized by measuring the chronological age-dependent decline of an array of different physiological functions.[26,27,31,48,54,55] In these measurements the maximum reserve capacity of physiological function is always determined. This is based on the fact that in the early phase of life there exists a certain amount of extra or reserve capacity over and above what is needed for survival that can be used in critical and emergency situations. As an individual grows older the reserve capacity steadily decreases until, at about the age of 40 years, there is no reserve capacity left. From that point onward a net decrease in physiological function capacity of the whole organism occurs. This is also about the age that individuals first really begin to "feel their age."

FIGURE 2 shows a typical plot of human physiological reserve capacity as a function of chronological age. Here it is seen that functional capacity increases steadily after birth, reaching a peak around sexual maturity or about 10 to 15 years of age. This is the ageat which an individual is essentially at the greatest state of youth. There is no significant plateau period where this maximal youth status remains constant. Instead, soon after the peak of health and maximum reserve capacity is reached, there is a steady, apparently linear decrease with age throughout the remaining period of an individual's life span.

I have defined the rate of this decrease in physiological functional capacity as the *aging rate* of the organism, in this case *Homo sapiens*. Of course this

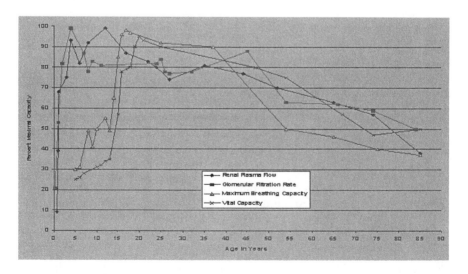

FIGURE 2. Typical plot of human physiological reserve capacity as a function of chronological age. (From Batitis and Sargent.[129] Reproduced by permission.)

slope is an average for a large group of people and certainly some individual differences are expected to exist.

Much research work over the past 50 years in gerontology has focused on understanding the nature or mechanisms of the processes leading to the well-characterized decline in physiological functional capacity. The goal here is that once we know what is causing aging or what the key processes are that are affected by aging, then we should be in a position to repair it. Yet today we still know very little about the primary mechanism(s) of aging and so essentially nothing about what or how to repair these problem(s).

There is another approach in reducing the effects of aging and increasing healthy and productive life span that has been proposed more than 20 years ago but is just now becoming increasingly popular.[8,9,11,56] This is to focus research on the processes controlling the rate of aging, which is represented by the slope of the curve shown in FIGURE 2. This approach is growing in popularity since considerable data now indicate that the mechanisms controlling aging rate may be much less complex than the aging processes they control.[32,57–60] The goal here would be to develop the means to decrease the rate at which humans presently, on average, lose normal body functions. This proposal is based on the observation that the slope of this curve is proportional to the life span of different mammalian species. Unfortunately this concept is based on very little data: we have data for the mouse, domestic animals, and some non-human primates, but not for primates. This points to the very serious problem of very little high-quality data available on the comparative biology of aging among primates, especially the chimpanzee.

AGING IS THE RESULT OF NORMAL DEVELOPMENTAL AND METABOLIC PROCESSES

To begin developing the means to control the rate of aging, there needs to be at least some theoretical basis of why aging exists, how it evolved, and how complex the processes might be that control rate of aging. Most of the theoretical work published in this area has been by evolutionary biologists and generally takes the view that aging has evolved because of the diminished importance chronologically old individuals have in reproductive value. This diminished importance is a result of individuals being steadily removed from the population because of random deaths from some type of environmental hazard. This key observation has led to the proposal that since there are always more individuals that are chronologically younger in populations living in their natural ecological niche, this population is favored to inherit the expression of genes that favor their survival even if these genes have decremental or aging effects when expressed at a higher chronological age. This then results in the accumulation of many different genes that have benefits when expressed in young individuals, but are less advantageous when expressed in older individuals. In fact, most genes in the genome may be involved in this type of aging process. This concept has been called the *antagonistic pleiotropic hypothesis* of aging.[61,62]

The prediction of this hypothesis is that aging of all living organisms occurs by this accumulation of antagonistic pleiotropic expressing genes. One very important consequence of this hypothesis is rarely pointed out: If the aging process of humans today is a result of expression of so many different genes having this pleiotropic nature, then it would appear to be impossible to alter this type of aging without changing essentially all the genes in the genome. But if this prediction is true, then how did longevity ever evolve in the first place and at such a rapid rate as is evident during the recent hominid ancestral descendent sequence leading to *Homo sapiens* over the past 10 million years? One answer is that longevity did not evolve and that it is essentially impossible to increase the life span of animals today because of the high genetic complexity of the antagonistic pleiotropic effect.[63–67]

This is not the place to debate these theories, but I would like to say that I have published an alternative view based on the concept that longevity rather than aging processes is what has evolved. My approach also has been of an evolutionary nature, but with the important distinction of starting with the evolution of the first forms of life rather than with metazoan animals.[8,68]

Most theoretical gerontologists in this field generally agree that aging is the result of normal development and metabolic processes and that is it is a byproduct of the very processes that are required for life to exist. This conclusion leads me to predict that there are no aging genes, but instead longevity genes.

Examples of four proposed developmental and metabolic processes that could be important contributors to aging are:

- byproducts of *development*, such as growth and sexual hormones;

- byproducts of *growth* and *size* determinants, such as growth factors limiting the size of internal organs;

- byproducts of *stress*, such as the adrenocorticoid hormones; and

- byproducts of *energy metabolism*, such as reactive oxygen and nitrogen species aand the glycation/glycoxidation AGE products.

I have proposed that two major strategies have evolved to postpone aging during the recent evolution of longevity in the primate species. The first strategy deals with all the age-producing pleiotropic acting genes, which I agree are likely to exist. These genes are associated with the genetic program of differentiation and development, where they are beneficial during the process of differentiation and development but become increasingly less beneficial and even toxic after the process of differentiation and development has been completed. I have proposed that by simply extending the genetic program of differentiation and development uniformly in time, the toxic effect of these genes are effectively eliminated for that period of extension of the genetic program.

Evidence for this occurrence is the remarkable extension or slowdown of the genetic program of differentiation and development. This is most obvious on observation of the remarkable positive correlation of age of sexual maturation with life span in mammalian species. Humans with the greatest life span have the oldest age of sexual maturity of the primate species. Thus, to further increase life span along the lines that have naturally evolved it appears to be essential to find the means to further reduce the present rate of human differentiation and development.

The second strategy deals with the toxic byproducts associated with energy metabolism. Here I am largely referring to the production of reactive oxygen and nitrogen species produced during the generation of energy within the mitochondria. These reactive oxygen and nitrogen species can react with most molecules within a cell and alter its structure and thus function. Perhaps most important is the possibility that these reactive species can alter the proper differentiated state of cells in an epigenetic manner. Thus it appears important for maintaining stability of proper cell function to reduce the amount of these reactive species as much as possible.

A number of different strategies have been discovered to do this. One strategy is simply to produce less-reactive species by reducing the metabolic rate of the organism or decreasing the leakage of these species from mitochondria. A second strategy is to increase the resistance of normal cellular constituents to reactive species attack. This is done for example by reduction of unsaturated fatty acids in lipids and metal/sulfur groups in proteins. A third strategy is to increase the concentration of antioxidants that remove the reactive species. A fourth strategy is to repair the damage, and a fifth is to degrade or turn over the damaged cellular structure before it interferes with normal cell function.

PRIMARY VS. NON-PRIMARY AGING PROCESSES

It is clear that the aging process itself is very complex since it appears to affect the organism at all levels of function. However it is important to realize that complex results do not necessarily mean their causes are of equal complexity. This is illustrated in FIGURE 3, where I propose two fundamental models illustrating the non-primary and the primary aging process models. In the non-primary model initial causes of aging at the initiation stage are of complexity equal to or greater than than the final phenotypic stage of aging. This model indicates the vast complexity of aging at all levels of organism function and strongly indicates how very difficult it may be to interfere or slow down aging at any level of function of the organism.

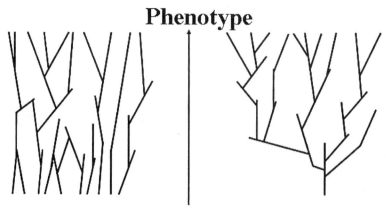

FIGURE 3. Two fundamental models of non-primary and primary aging process.

The primary model has equal level of complexity at the phenotypic level but proposed the existence of one or a few primary initial causes of the cascade process of aging. This model emphasizes the important possibility that, in spite of the vast complexity of the aging process itself, theoretically the root of the propagation of the aging process could in principle be very simple. Thus, if the primary model is correct, then the problem of controlling aging rate would be a magnitude of order less complex.

THE BREAKTHROUGH: THE HUMAN AGES AT HALF THE RATE OF THE CHIMPANZEE BUT HAS A REMARKABLY SIMILAR BIOLOGY

It is well known that different species have different life spans, as is clearly evident by the various domestic animals with which we are familiar. However, in 1971, when I was examining the life spans of primate species I was struck by the wide range of life spans that existed within closely related species and particularly the primates.

Examples are shown in TABLE 1, where the human clearly has the greatest life span (of about 120 years) followed by the chimpanzee with about 60 years. The shortest lifespan was that of the tree shrew, which has a lifespan of about 8 years.

What I found amazing was that these species were all very closely related to one another, having common ancestors with substantial differences in life

TABLE 1. Maximal life span potentials for some primate species

Species and subspecies	Representative	Years
Homo sapiens	Man	120
Pan troglodytes	Chimpanzee	60
Cebus capuncinus	Capuchin	40
Galago senegalensis	Galago	25
Tarsius syrichta	Tarsier	12
Urogale everetti	Tree shrew	8

NOTE: Taken by permission from Cutler.[68]

span. Here the most exciting example was between human and chimpanzee, having a common ancestor only about 5 million years ago, a high genomic sequence identity, and remarkably similar biology. These data immediately indicated that the biological basis determining general health maintenance may not be nearly as complex as has been proposed.

For example, it was generally thought that aging is a wear-and-tear processes similar to what we observe in most every thing surrounding us, such as the automobile. Humans being unusually long-lived were viewed in this wear-and-tear model as the Mercedes Benz class of primates: they have superior design and engineering and are made up of better, longer-lasting, and stronger parts. Thus to get a Mercedes Benz to last even longer and go more miles before it wore out required essentially that the entire car be reengineered. So it was also thought for humans that increasing human life span was not possible because of the high complexity of the job of fixing everything. Usually this argument is followed by the comment that we should all be happy with the life span we have.

Yet I now find evidence of a two-fold difference in life span and aging rate between human and chimpanzee, while their parts and design are essentially the same! One popular explanation of how new and different species evolved is that it is largely a result of differences in the timing and degree of expression of a common set of genes and not the evolution of new genes. This model fits well in explaining at least the morphological difference between human and chimpanzee. For example, on comparing the skeleton of these two species, we see that the design is clearly the same where both species have the same bones. This is evident by being able to map or transform the entire skeleton of an adult human to the skeleton of a chimpanzee. The design is clearly the same and only the size (length and width) of the individual bones are different. Could it be that similar design exists throughout the entire composition of the bodies of humans and chimpanzees and that the only key difference is the timing and degrees of expression of a common set of genes?

Perhaps the most exciting part of this discovery was the realization that if this model of species evolution was correct, then it implied that humans and chimpanzees also shared common genes that controlled the rate of aging, where the only difference was the timing and degree of their expression. If this was true, then further increase of human life span was possible through changes in expression of these common genes and nothing new in terms of new genes needs to be invented.[3] Since the percent difference in genomic sequence between human and chimpanzee had been estimated to be 98%, it appears that these common genes controlling life span were relatively few in number.[8]

GENETIC COMPLEXITY GOVERNING HUMAN LONGEVITY

It has generally been thought that the aging process and the processes controlling aging rate are extraordinary complex. Yet there have been few studies reported to obtain reasonable complexity estimates. The question I wanted to focus on was just how complex genetically were the processes controlling aging rate in human? I discovered a way of doing this by studying how fast life span evolved along the hominid ancestral descendent sequence leading to the modern *Homo sapiens*.[8,9] FIGURE 4 shows the evolution of human lifespan over the past 1.5 million years. Estimates of life span were made using the Sacher brain/body allometric equation.

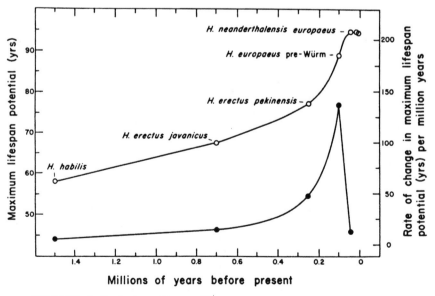

FIGURE 4. Evolution of human life span over the past 1.5 million years.

Results of these studies indicated that life span increased 14 years per 100,000 years in hominids about 100,000 years ago. This rate suggests that a genetic complexity of less than 250 genes could be involved. These genes were defined as *longevity-determinant genes*. From this point onward, the field of gerontology has dramatically changed since for the first time there was now a reasonably sound rationale to believe that the human aging process is subject to control by relatively few genetic or biochemical interventions.

THE UNIQUELY HIGH LIFE-SPAN ENERGY POTENTIAL OF THE HUMAN

Now that we had a rational basis for believing that few genes may be involved in the control of the human rate of aging, we needed to know more about what their function might be to help us in their identification. So we set out to search for key genetic, biochemical, and physiological differences between human and chimpanzee that may have an impact on the aging rate.

It is well known that the human has the longest life span of all primate species and most mammalian species. Yet we also found that the human consumes more energy over its life span than do other species. This is shown in FIGURE 5, where life span (MLSP) is plotted against specific metabolic rate (SMR) for many different mammalian species.

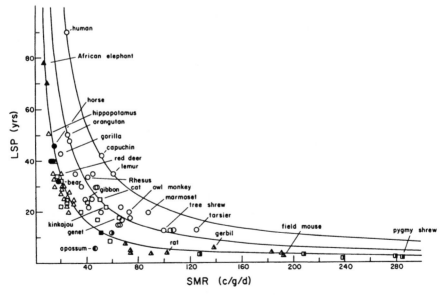

FIGURE 5. Life span (LSP) plotted against specific metabolic rate (SMR) for different mammalian species.

In this figure the data appear to separate into three curves. These curves follow the hyperbolic function: LEP = (MLSP) (SMR) where LEP is life-span energy potential.

The top curve contains data for only the human, lemur, and the capuchin with a LEP value of about 781 kc/g. The middle curve contains all other primate species having a LEP (life energy potential) value of about 458 kc/g. The lower curve contains all other mammalian species having a LEP value of about 220 kc/g.

These data indicate that the human is unique in being able to consume more energy over its life span. On the basis of this result, longevity-determinant genes would then be predicted to include higher expression of genes involved in protecting human cells against energy metabolism. This suggests an important role of free radicals related to energy metabolism as a cause of aging and of protective processes such as antioxidants and DNA repair processes as determinants of longevity.

SPECIFIC AGE-RELATED HUMAN DISEASES ASSOCIATED WITH OXIDATIVE STRESS AND INFLAMMATION

Since we now had an independent rationale for considering oxidative stress as a potential cause of aging, we examined the many different age-related diseases to determine whether they may have an oxidative stress–causative component. The results of this search are shown in TABLE 2.

To my surprise it appeared that many if not most of the common age-dependent diseases of humans do have potential oxidative stress as either a primary or secondary cause and/or an aggravating or propagation factor.[1,69–84] Thus these data also independently support oxidative stress as being a possible important component of the aging process itself.

COMPARATIVE STUDIES OF OXIDATIVE STRESS AS A PRIMARY CAUSE OF AGING

Our experiments at this point have suggested that the proposed longevity-determinant genes may be involved in controlling oxidative stress levels in tissues. Thus we now know what type of genes or biochemistry to examine to further test this hypothesis.

Superoxide Dismutase

Our first experiments were to measure the enzymatic activity of superoxide dismutase (SOD) in tissues of animals as a function of their life span.[85] Our

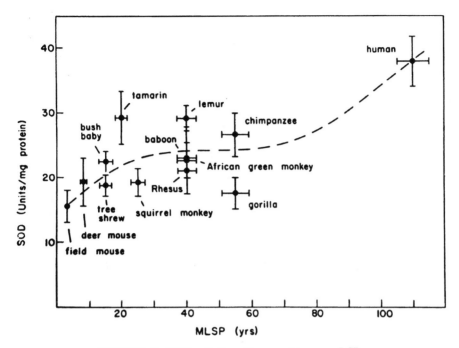

FIGURE 6. SOD activity with respect to mean LSP.

prediction was that if SOD genes were one of the longevity-determinant genes, we would expect a higher expression of this gene with increased life span of the primate species and in particular higher expression in the same tissue in humans compared to chimpanzees.

In these comparative studies we chose to focus on the primate species since they are most closely related to the human and these are the species in which we had originated studies that suggested these experiments. Results of the SOD experiments are shown in FIGURES 6 and 7.

In these initial studies we measured total liver SOD activity (SOD1 + SOD2). FIGURE 6 shows that SOD activity does in general increase with increased life span, having the lowest activity in mouse and the highest in humans. Also, it was clear that liver SOD activity was greater in the human than in the chimpanzee. But there was not any significant correlation in the other non-human primate species.

We then realized that our comparison analysis was incorrect. What we should be measuring is the relative level of SOD protection that existed per amount of superoxide free radical generated. Since we had no means at that time to measure endogenous production of the superoxide radical, we made the assumption that it would be in proportion to the specific metabolic rate of

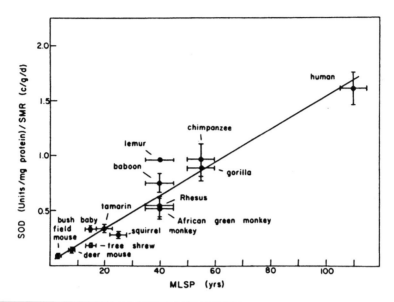

FIGURE 7. SOD activity with respect to mean LSP.

the tissue. That is, the amount of oxygen used by the tissue would be proportional to the amount of superoxide radical produced. Thus. we next normalized our data, now plotting SOD per SMR as a function of life span. Results of this analysis are shown in FIGURE 7, indicating a remarkable linear relationship for all species used in the study.

It is also of interest to note here that these data also show that the LEP value of the species used in this study is directly proportional to the SOD value of their tissues. Thus we have another confirmation of our previous LEP studies, suggesting that one reason why LEP value is so high in humans is because they have extra protection against the toxic byproducts of energy metabolism. This SOD study confirmed the theoretically based prediction and it represents the first time an enzyme activity has ever been shown to be associated with the life span of any species. These data have also since been confirmed independently in another laboratory.[86]

Finally, it is important to note that a number of years after this study it was reported that the generation of the superoxide radical is not proportional just to SMR, but instead decreases with increased life span of the animal.[87–92] So if this is true, then the correlation we have reported would be even more striking, indicating both an increase in SOD and a decrease in superoxide radical leakiness from mitochondria as being important longevity determinants. Genes controlling free radical leakiness may involve the uncoupling genes of mitochondrial membranes, and we are presently checking that possibility.

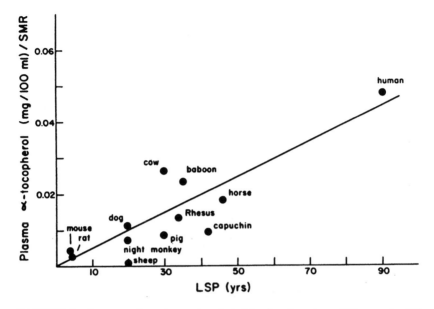

FIGURE 8. Concentration of tocopherols in blood as function of life span in different species.

Tocopherols and Carotenoids

We next measured the concentration of the tocopherols (vitamin E) and the carotenoids in blood as a function of life span in different species.[12] These data are shown in FIGURES 8 and 9, respectively.

For both vitamin E and the carotenoids we find a strong positive correlation of their concentration in serum with life span, again supporting a possibly important role of antioxidants in reducing the aging rate of mammalian species.

Although tocopherols are generally thought to be important in fertility and most perhaps afford protection against oxidative stress, new functions are being discovered not involving these processes. So the possible role of high tocopherol in promoting human longevity is still an open question. Of course, more data on different tissues are required to confirm these pilot studies.

Carotenoids are generally thought to be important only as a precursor to vitamin A, and here the presence of carotenoids would be expected largely in liver tissue. The high levels found in all tissues of the human has long been a puzzle and is often explained as a human defect. Carotenoids have now been shown to induce other antioxidant genes, so again, as with the tocopherols, the role carotenoids may have in promoting human longevity may go beyond their properties as an antioxidant.

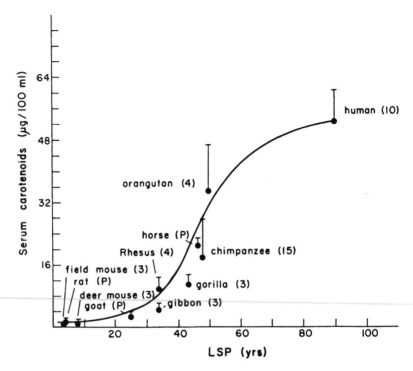

FIGURE 9. Concentration of carotenoids in blood as function of life span in different species.

What genes are possibly responsible for controlling the serum levels of these antioxidants is not clear. There are now some data indicating that tocopherol serum levels are regulated to some extent by active transport mechanisms, possibly the newly discovered transporting tocopherol proteins. There are enzymes in the intestine that specifically cleave and degrade the carotenoids, and the activity of these enzymes is unusually low in the human.

Uric Acid

Although uric acid is generally thought to be a waste product of purine metabolism, it has now been shown to have antioxidant properties. Given its high concentration in human serum, it is the dominant antioxidant. Thus it was important to see whether serum levels of uric acid were associated with the life span of mammalian species. These data are shown in FIGURE 10, indicating a strong positive correlation of increased concentration with increased life span.[93]

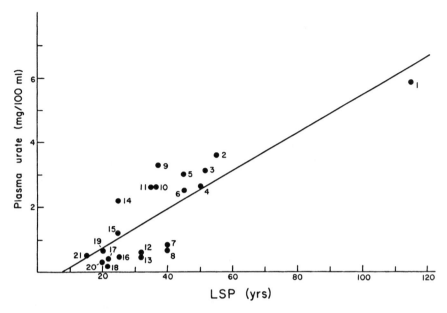

FIGURE 10. Plasma urate levels as a function of LSP. 1, human; 2, chimpanzee; 3, orangutan; 4, gorilla; 5, gibbon; 6, capuchin; 7, macaque; 8, baboon; 9, spider monkey; 10, Siamang gibbon; 11, wooly monkey; 12, langur; 13, grivet; 14, tamarin; 15, squirrel monkey; 16, night monkey; 17, potto; 18, patas; 19, galago; 20, howler monkey; 21, tree shrew. Correlation coefficient line is $r = 0.85$, where P is less than or equal to 0.001. (Taken in part from Cutler.[13] Reprinted by permission.)

The mechanisms leading to this increase involve the activity of the uricase enzyme and transport properties of uric acid in the kidney. Of interest, uricase appears to have steadily decreased as life span increased, and its activity is completely absent in the human. The knockout of uricase appears to have occurred at about the time humans also lost the ability to synthesize vitamin C. Some have speculated that uric acid is a safer antioxidant than vitamin C and as a metal chelator it acts to protect vitamin C.

Finally it is known that uric acid is a methyl xanthine-like caffeine and that people who have high urate levels tend to excel at what they attempt, despite having modest talents. Individuals with high uric acid levels are often found as heads of companies or chairmen of departments.

Thus the evolution of higher uric acid levels may have occurred as a result of downregulation of the uric acid gene, and the benefits may have been the lowering of oxidative stress and the stimulus of activities to succeed. The blood concentration of urate is close to the maximum in humans where higher levels would seriously increase the incidence of gout. So it appears that the strategem of increasing urate acid to increase life span in the human is not likely to be an option any longer.

TOTAL ANTIOXIDANT CAPACITY OF SERUM
AS A FUNCTION OF LIFE SPAN

There are many more specific antioxidants, such as the polyphenols, that could be measured separately. It is possible that the positive correlations we have found are special cases and do not reflect the general rule. So I developed a new technique to measure total antioxidant capacity of the serum to test the hypothesis that increased protection of tissues from oxidative stress leads to a longer and healthier life span.

The name of this new assay was oxygen radical absorption capacity assay or the ORAC assay.[94] We applied this assay to measure total antioxidant in serum samples taken from different mammalian species. Results are shown in FIGURE 11.

We found that human serum had the greatest ORAC value and that in general the ORAC value of serum increased with an increase in life span of primate species. These data indicate not only that there is an increase in tocopherols, carotenoids, and uric acid with increased life span, with the human having the highest value in all these cases, but also that total antioxidant capacity of serum is greatest in the human compared to the shorter-lived primates.

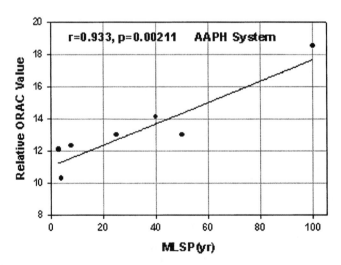

FIGURE 11. ORAC value in serum samples from different mammalian species.

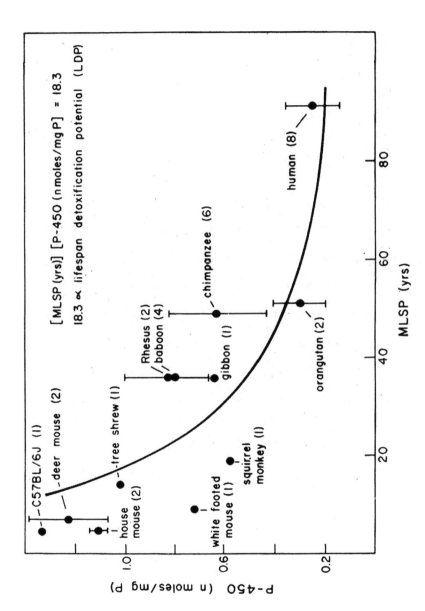

FIGURE 12. P450 activity as a function of life span of different mammalian species.

Cytochrome P450 System

The cytochrome P450 system has a protective role in the detoxification of many of the toxic components of food in an animal's diet. So we asked whether the human was unique in having unusually high levels of this detoxification system. This was determined by measuring total P450 activity in liver tissue as a function of life span of different mammalian species, again with an emphasis on primate species.[16] Results of this study are shown in FIGURE 12.

Results were surprising: We found a decrease, rather than an increase, in P450 with increased life span. However, on closer study, we found that the P450 system generates hydrogen peroxide, which can be converted to the hydroxyl radical. So here it appears that we have an example of *decreasing* a source of oxidative stress rather than *increasing* protection against the free radicals produced.

We also found a similar decrease in liver of the antioxidants catalase and glutathione peroxidase. Both of these antioxidant enzymes are active in removal of hydrogen. We speculated that this result is consistent with the lowering of P450 and hydrogen production, decreasing the need for the presence of hydrogen-peroxide protective enzymes.

Autoxidation Capacity of Tissues

The results discussed so far supported the hypothesis that oxidative stress is an important factor in determining the aging rate of a species. Yet we needed a better global test of the net sensitivity of whole tissues against oxidative reaction. To accomplish this goal we decided to measure the rate of peroxidation or autoxidation of whole-tissue homogenates.[14] The rate of this reaction would be dependent on many different factors. These would include the sensitivity of the tissue homogenates to peroxidation reactions—that is, their innate peroxidizability. It would also depend on the presence of antioxidants, particularly chain-breaking antioxidants such as vitamin E and trace metals, which are known to catalyse such reactions. There are also likely to be many other factors that affect the sensitivity of tissues to autoxidation reactions.

In this experiment we simply incubated the homogenate tissue (brain in this example) in air, and by taking samples periodically, we measured the kinetics of the autoxidation reaction. Peroxidation was measured using the thiobarbituric acid assay (often known as the TBARM assay) on five brain-tissue samples of equal amount for five different species having wide differences in life span. The original data of this now classic experiment are shown in FIGURE 13.

The results of this experiment show the time-dependent accumulation of peroxidation products for five different species. The rate of increase is greatest for the mouse and the total amount of peroxidation product in this species

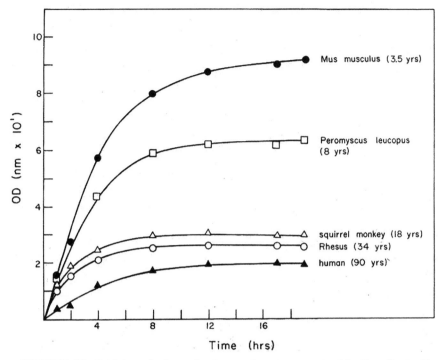

FIGURE 13. Initial results from classic experiment concerning kinetics of autoxidation of brain homogenate.

was also greatest. Similar results were obtained for the other four species, where, for increasing life span, the brain tissue was increasingly more resistant to autoxidation. Most importantly, it is clear that the human brain samples were most resistant to spontaneous peroxidation reactions.

These experiments were repeated many times and on many different species and tissues, and the results were always the same. With increased life span, the rate and total amount or percent of tissue peroxidation decreased with the increased life span of the donor animal.

The results represent some of the strongest support for the general importance of oxidative stress as a cause of aging and for the notion that an important control of oxidative stress is the sensitivity of the tissue to peroxidation reactions. This conclusion is more evident when the data are further analysed, showing that the major variable was the percentage of the brain sample that was peroxidizable. Since peroxidation is largely a result of lipid peroxidation reactions, these results suggest that the lipids making up the composition of brain have a lower percentage of unsaturated fatty acids in the longer-lived species. This prediction was later confirmed by actual measurements of the composition of lipids taken from different species.[95–104] The peroxidizability of the sample was calculated from the fatty acid composition profile of the samples, and the results showed that the peroxidizability index decreased significantly with increased life span.

The fatty acid composition of lipids is controlled by several common genes in all mammalian species and so it is predicted that a change in the relative degree of their expression will explain the difference in composition. What is particularly interesting here is that human lipids have the greatest resistance to lipid peroxidation as a result of a decrease in unsaturated fatty acids, but the fluidity of the membranes of the tissue remains unchanged.

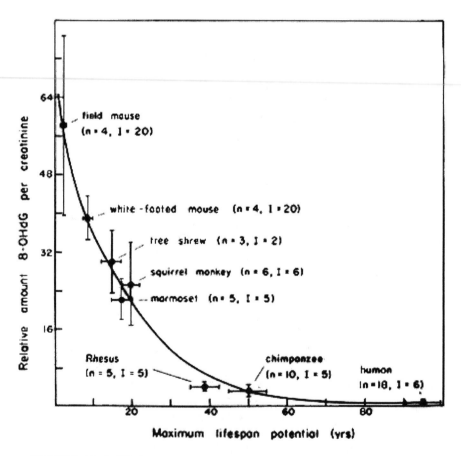

FIGURE 14. 8-OHdG per unit of creatinine in urine samples taken from different species as a function of age.

OXIDATIVE DNA DAMAGE AS A FUNCTION OF LIFE SPAN

As part of our working hypothesis it was predicted that the steady state of oxidative damage of DNA would decrease with increasing life span. We did not have the technique at the time to test this hypothesis, but after we informed Dr. Bruce Ames of our planned experiments, he was able to carry out the experiments himself.[105,106] We were later able to confirm and expand his original results.[107-109] These data are shown in FIGURE 14, which shows the amount of 8-OHdG per creatinine unit in urine samples taken from different species as a function of age.

The results clearly show that with increased life span of the species, the amount of 8-OHdG per unit of creatinine in the urine sample steadily decreases with increase of life span. This is exactly what was predicted in my original paper on this subject in 1972. In our studies we had evidence that oxidative damage was greatest at a very young age (1 to 5 years old), was lowest in middle life, and then begin to increase again in the last third of the life span. On examining the time course of DNA damage, we found that with increasing life span the percentage of damage present at very young ages of different species dramatically decreased. These data need confirmation, but, if correct, they indicate that the stage of life when oxidative stress is greatest is early life and that later, after a long latent period, the adult and older individual begin to suffer the consequence. Of course, if that species were living in its natural ecological niche, it would have likely died from natural predators rather than from cancer or other consequences of DNA damage.

DIRECT TEST OF THE OXIDATIVE STRESS HYPOTHESIS OF LONGEVITY

So far all I have presented are correlative data and not the results of cause-and-effect type of experiments. One of the best tests of the hypothesis that oxidative stress is important to aging and that antioxidants play a role is to create transgenic mice that have a higher-expressed antioxidant coding gene. Several laboratories have done these experiments and I am pleased to say they were all successful. These transgenic experiments include *Drosophila* and mice. Two mouse experiments are summarized here:

- Mice transgenic for the *thioredoxin* or the *catalase* genes have a *greater* resistance to oxidative stress and about a 25 to 30 percent increase in mean and maximal life span (results from the research groups of Dr. Junji Yodoi and of Dr. George Martin presented elsewhere in this volume).

- Mice with a mutation in the p66 adapter protein gene have a greater resistance to oxidative stress and about a 25 to 30 percent increase in life span (Dr. Pier G. Pelicci's research group).

Of particular interest is the thioredoxin (trx-1) transgenic mouse on a C57BL/6 mouse strain background that showed a 25% increase in life expectancy and life span.[110–116] Similar results have been reported by Dr. George Martin for a catalase transgenic mouse strain on a mouse strain with the same genetic background.[111] A mutation in the p66 adapter protein was also shown to increase resistance in oxidative stress and to increase life span by 25–30 percent.[117–120]

HOW DOES OXIDATIVE STRESS CAUSE AGING? THE DYSDIFFERENTIATION HYPOTHESIS OF AGING

Usually it is thought that the reactive oxygen and nitrogen species cause aging by the damage they produce. Usually the focus is DNA damage, but oxidized proteins also are likely to be important as are oxidized organelles such as mitochondria. The general idea is that with increasing age this damage steadily increases throughout the body of the organism (both inside and outside cells). This results in fewer functional proteins (inside and outside the cells) and fewer functional cellular organelles and then finally fewer cells. The result is a steady decrease in the net functional capacity of the organism with increasing age.

The problem I find with this scenario (which is really the old wear-and-tear hypothesis) is that there is little evidence of such large amounts of damage, except at the last stages of the life span. So there is no good correlation of the well-established linear decline in physiological functions with increase in oxidative damage in cells. In fact, cells from middle-aged mice have little oxidative damage, but they certainly show the signs of being old.

Aging is largely a result of the natural limitation of the genetic apparatus of a cell to be able to maintain over time the proper state of differentiation of its cells.[2,121–128] The proper state of differentiation in cells is taken to be that when the program of differentiation and development was completed.

Very little is known of what mechanisms act to stabilize the proper differentiated state of cells, but oxidatively mediated alterations of regulatory proteins could certainly alter large transcription profile patterns of cells in an epigenetic manner. This hypothesis implies that aging is a result of the same type of epigenetically mediated changes in gene expression profiles that naturally occurred during the normal differentiation and developmental program. Thus it would be predicted that cells making up a long-lived organism would be found to be more stable in maintaining the proper differentiated state of its cell than would be cells making up a shorter-lived species.

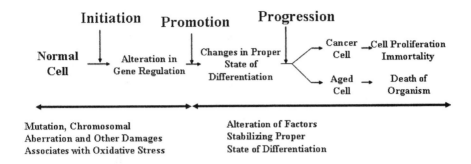

FIGURE 15. Model of aging dysdifferentiated cells in cancer.

Oxidative stress comes into this picture because I predicted that the genetic apparatus of the cell is by far a more sensitive target for reactive oxygen species than other cells targets. Here small oxidatively mediated types of damage could have far reaching consequences in cell function. Another aspect of this model of aging is that the age-dependent increase of cancer is readily explained since cancer is simply a special case of an aged dysdifferentiated cell. These points are summarized below and in FIGURE 15

Hypotheses for how oxidative stress causes aging are:

- Aging is largely a result of *epigenetically* based *dysdifferentiation* processes and is responsible for the linear age-dependent decline in physiological functions.

- The major determinants of aging rate or life span are those processes that act to *protect* and *stabilize* the proper differentiated state of cells making up the organism.

- Oxidative stress acts to *accelerate* the epigenetically based dysdifferentiation processes.

- Those processes that act to *control oxidative stress* also control in part the *rate of dysdifferentiation* and thus the aging rate or life span of the animal.

FIGURE 15 presents a model proposing that aging and cancer have common mechanisms of causation and control. Similar models can be constructed based more on epigenetically mediated alterations of gene expression.

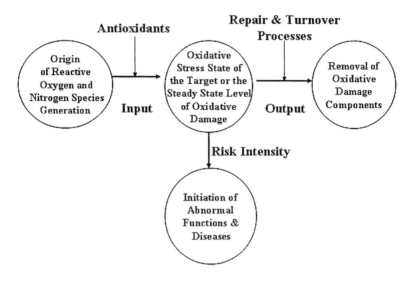

FIGURE 16. Rationale of tests to be used to assess intensity of risk for high levels of oxidative stress.

DEVELOPING THE STRATEGY AND MEANS TO DETERMINE THE OXIDATIVE STRESS STATUS OF HUMAN INDIVIDUALS

The previous information provides some of the rationale for the importance that measuring oxidative stress status of an individual would have in aid of optimizing health and longevity. The question now is: Will our present knowledge and technology allow us to do this now? And if so, then how?

FIGURE 16 presents a model of oxidative stress and risk to disease. It illustrates a rationale of what tests should be included to best assess the risk intensity of poor health as a result of high levels of oxidative stress.

The goal is to assess the steady-state level of oxidative damage in the whole body, which is considered to be proportional to the risk of age-related diseases. This figure points out that the steady-state level of oxidative stress is determined by relative rates of damage input and damage removal. These parameters are difficult to assess, however, so, instead, antioxidant and oxidative damage levels are obtained from a blood and urine sample to estimate the person's oxidative stress status.

OPTIMIZATION OF HEALTH OF AN INDIVIDUAL
BY A MINIMIZATION OF OXIDATIVE STRESS STATUS

As briefly reviewed here, much evidence exists that oxidative stress plays a role as a risk factor in many age-dependent diseases and is possibly also involved as a key determinant of how fast the general aging process proceeds. Since the major causes of death are the age-dependent diseases, it appears reasonable to predict that lowering an individual's oxidative stress status would result in decreasing the risk of incurring these diseases. Since we know of no benefit of oxidative stress or of the damage it represents, minimization of oxidative stress is expected to provide some general health benefits. The big question is how to do it.

Our strategy has been to measure an array of parameters related to oxidative stress as well as a number of clinical tests in an individual using a serum and urine sample. The results of these tests are also presented on a percentile basis so that different assays with different units of measurement can be summarized. From this information we will determine both the net level of steady-state oxidative damage on the one hand and the net levels of antioxidant protection on the other. This information would be used by a physician to determine whether the individual is under an abnormal level of oxidative stress and, if so, how best to treat the condition. Several follow-up tests are likely to be needed for the physician to finally arrive at what works best for the patient to achieve a minimum oxidative stress status. This is illustrated in FIGURE 17.

Factors that govern oxidative stress status are listed in TABLE 3.

These factors are classified into three components: hereditary, dietary, and environmental. There is little an individual can do about heredity, but dietary and environment factors are under an individual's control to lower his or her oxidative stress status.

An important basic concept here is the optimization of health through a feedback loop as illustrated in FIGURE 17.

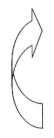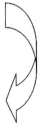

Assessment of General
Health & Health
Maintenance Status

Intervention Therapies

FIGURE 17.

The major problem to be solved in developing the oxidative stress profiling protocol is to determine whether it is possible to measure reliably the oxidative stress status of an individual so that it can provide meaningful data upon which the physician can act. This problem is particularly difficult since the procedure must be noninvasive and thus limited to a urine and blood sample. An additional serious complication is human biological variability, which can be substantial, depending on diet and exercise as well as on other factors, such as the variation that can result when the same tests are taken on different days.

A secondary problem is, of course, in developing biochemical assays to measure oxidative damage and antioxidants that are highly reproducible on the same urine or blood sample. Reliability of the biochemical tests measuring oxidative damage products in urine and serum samples was increased by using several different assays measuring the same type of damage by different procedures. We typically had a redundancy factor of two to three for each test. In addition, we compared these redundant tests to determine how well they correlated to each other.

In general, our tests had a coefficent of variation (CV) value range of 5–10% and individual bioavailability was about double this value or 10–20%. Thus, overall reproducibility of tests was in the range of 15–30%, which was sufficient, overall, for practical use. However, we are continuing to try to reduce this variability.

THE KRONOS SCIENCE LABORATORY REPORT

A typical report from the Kronos Laboratory of some of the assays used is assessing the oxidative stress status of an individual is shown in FIGURES 18 and 19. In general, we find an inverse correlation of oxidative damage with antioxidant levels, as indicated by the point in FIGURE 20. This type of analysis plotting oxidative damage against antioxidant protection provides important information as to how best to treat individuals having high levels of oxidative stress.

A summary of preliminary results obtained with patients is as follows:

- Individuals having oxidative stress levels *substantially greater than normal reference levels* show the best response to therapeutic measures to lower this stress.

- We have been *unable* to bring any individual to the point of having *substantially below-normal levels* of oxidative stress even after supplementation with mega-doses of antioxidants.

- A common cause of excessive oxidative stress in men was found to be high tissue levels of *iron*.

Oxidative Stress

Assay	Flag	U.S. Reference Ranges				International Reference Ranges			
		Value	Kronos Optimal	Normal	Units	Value	Kronos Optimal	Normal	Units
OXIDATIVE STRESS DAMAGE FACTORS									
DIRECT DAMAGE									
PEROXIDES AQ SER*		8.5	0.0-5.54	0.84-10.2	umol/L	8.5	0.0-5.54	0.84-10.2	umol/L
INDIRECT DAMAGE									
COPPER		1,250	700-900	498-1,945	ug/L	19.7	11-14.2	7.85-30.7	umol/L
FERRITIN		88	24-150	24-336	ng/mL	88	24-150	24-336	ug/L
GLUCOSE		89	60-95	74-118	mg/dL	4.94	3.33-5.27	4.11-6.55	mmol/L
HEMOGLOBIN A1C		5.2	4.0-5.0	4.0-6.0	%	5.2	4.0-5.0	4.0-6.0	%
IRON		85	28-99	45-182	ug/dL	15.2	5.01-17.7	8.06-32.6	umol/L
IRON BIND % SAT		27	10-36	10-36	%	27	10-36	10-36	%

FIGURE 18. Typical report from Kronos Laboratory of assays used in assessing oxidative stress.

Assay	Flag	U.S. Reference Ranges				International Reference Ranges			
		Value	Kronos Optimal	Normal	Units	Value	Kronos Optimal	Normal	Units
OXIDATIVE STRESS PROTECTON FACTORS									
ENDOGENOUS									
ALBUMIN		4.2	3.8-4.6	3.5-4.8	g/dL	42	38-46	35-48	g/L
BILIRUBIN, DIRECT		0.1	0.1-0.5	0.1-0.5	mg/dL	1.71	1.71-8.55	1.71-8.55	umol/L
BILIRUBIN, TOTAL		0.7	0.4-2.0	0.4-2.0	mg/dL	12	6.84-34.2	6.84-34.2	umol/L
CERULOPLASMIN		32	20-36	25-63	mg/dL	32	20-36	25-63	mg/dL
GLUTATHIONE*		8.8	6.0-10	2.0-12	uM	8.8	6.0-10	2.0-12	uM
CYSTEINE*		300	275-475	245-501	umol/L	300	275-475	245-501	umol/L
CYSTEINYLGLYCINE*		60	34-82	34-82	umol/L	60	34-82	34-82	umol/L
UIBC		230	254-382	126-382	ug/dL	41.2	45.5-68.4	22.6-68.4	umol/L
TIBC CALCULATED		315	370-478	261-478	ug/dL	56.4	66.3-85.6	46.7-85.6	umol/L
TOTAL THIOLS*		377	448-578	318-578	umol/L	377	448-578	318-578	umol/L
URIC ACID	L	4.7	6.8-8.7	4.8-8.7	mg/dL	0.277	0.401-0.513	0.283-0.513	mmol/L
EXOGENOUS									
ASCORBATE(VIT C)*		10	17-28	5.0-28	ug/mL	568	965-1,590	284-1,590	umol/L
COENZYME Q10 *		1.0	0.85-1.2	0.5-1.2	ug/mL	1.16	0.984-1.39	0.579-1.39	umol/L
SELENIUM		220	158-360	137-360	ug/L	2.79	2.0-4.56	1.73-4.56	umol/L

FIGURE 18. *Continued.*

CAROTENOIDS

Analyte	Value	Range	Range	Units	Value	Range	Range	Units
CAROTENE, ALPHA*	99	40-200	20-400	ng/mL	0.184	0.074-0.372	0.037-0.744	umol/L
CAROTENE, BETA*	400	200-600	50-710	ng/mL	0.744	0.372-1.12	0.093-1.32	umol/L
CRYPTOXANTHIN, BETA*	80	70-200	5.0-200	ng/mL	145	127-362	9.05-362	nmol/L
LUTEIN*	128	125-400	40-600	ng/mL	0.225	0.22-0.704	0.07-1.06	umol/L
LYCOPENE*	142	180-350	10-350	ng/mL	0.264	0.335-0.651	0.019-0.651	umol/L
RETINOL*	480	850-1,300	400-1,300	ng/mL	1,675	2,967-4,537	1,396-4,537	nmol/L
RETINYL PALMITATE*	19	16-27	5.0-27	ng/mL	0.034	0.029-0.049	0.009-0.049	umol/L
ZEAXANTHIN*	40	80-150	10-150	ng/mL	70.3	141-264	17.6-264	nmol/L

TOCOPHEROL

Analyte	Value	Range	Range	Units	Value	Range	Range	Units
TOCOPHEROL, ALPHA*	15	14.8-22.4	7.2-22.4	ug/mL	34.8	34.4-52	16.7-52	umol/L
TOCOPHEROL, DELTA*	0.07	0.13-0.2	0.05-0.2	ug/mL	0.174	0.323-0.497	0.124-0.497	umol/L
TOCOPHEROL, GAMMA*	1.3	1.15-2.2	0.1-2.2	ug/mL	3.12	2.76-5.28	0.24-5.28	umol/L

* This test was developed and its performance characteristics determined by Kronos Science Laboratories, Inc. It has not been cleared or approved by the U.S. Food and Drug Administration.

Green areas on bar graphs represent the Kronos range for optimal health. Yellow areas on bar graphs represent the normal reference range. Red areas on bar graphs represent value ranges outside of the normal reference range.

© 2003 Kronos Science, Patent Pending

CollectedDate	Patient ID		Patient Name	Accession Number
03/18/04	RF-4384	II- 1	REPORT, MALE	H4020

FIGURE 18. *Continued.*

Lipograph ™

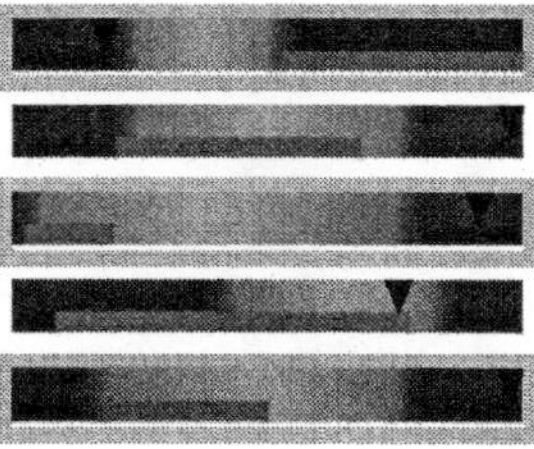

Assay	Flag	Value	Kronos Optimal Range	Normal Range	Units
NCEP ATP III PRIMARY LIPID PANEL					
HDL	L	38	65-107	40-70	mg/dL
LDL (DIRECT)	H	114	50-90	50-100	mg/dL
VLDL	H	36	1.0-8.0	1.0-30	mg/dL
CHOLESTEROL (TOTAL)		188	110-190	150-200	mg/dL
TRIGLYCERIDES	H	196	35-100	35-160	mg/dL

FIGURE 19. Typical report from Kronos Laboratory of assays used in assessing oxidative stress.

LDL LIPOPROTEIN SUBFRACTIONS

VLDL	H	36	1.0-8.0	1.0-30	mg/dL
IDL 1		12.5	7.0-10.5	7.0-14	mg/dL
IDL 2	L	2.09	4.5-6.75	4.5-9.0	mg/dL
IDL 3	H	25.1	8.0-12	8.0-16	mg/dL
LDL 1	H	40.5	19-28.5	19-38	mg/dL
LDL 2	H	29.4	9.5-14.3	9.5-19	mg/dL
LDL 3	H	4.38	2.0-3.0	2.0-4.0	mg/dL
LDL 4		0.0	0.0-0.0	0.0-0.0	mg/dL

LDL PATTERN PROFILE

MEAN LDL PARTICLE SIZE		269	270-276	262-271	Å

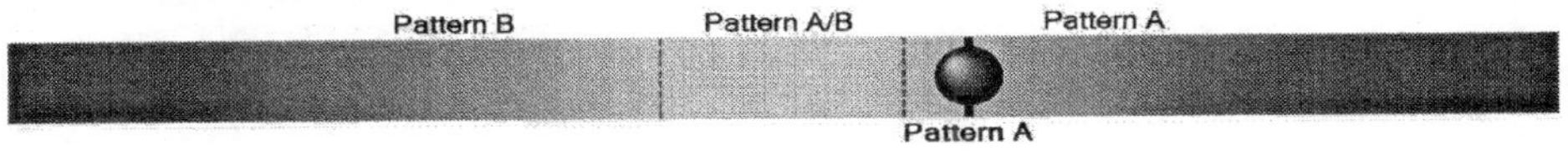

Pattern B   Pattern A/B   Pattern A

Pattern A

FIGURE 19. *Continued.*

HDL LIPOPROTEIN SUBFRACTIONS

HDL 1 (HDL 2b) *	L	2.28	11.9-25.3	10-25.3	mg/dL
HDL 2 *	L	7.98	12.2-23.1	10-23.1	mg/dL
HDL 3 *		27.7	26.5-37.8	20-37.8	mg/dL

OTHER CARDIOVASCULAR RISK FACTORS

HOMOCYSTEINE	H	10.5	3.0-7.5	3.0-12	umol/L
CRP-HS		0.5	0.0-0.2	0.0-0.25	mg/dL
LP(a)		5.0	0.0-10	0.0-79.1	mg/dL

REFERENCE RANGES: CAUCASIAN/ASIAN [<48mg/dL] HISPANIC[<13mg/dL] AFRICAN AND DESCENDANTS[<72mg/dL] NATIVE AMERICAN[<35mg/dL]

* This test was developed and its performance characteristics determined by Kronos Science Laboratories, Inc. It has not been cleared or approved by the U.S. Food and Drug Administration.

Green areas on bar graphs represent the Kronos range for optimal health. Yellow areas on bar graphs represent the normal reference range. Red areas on bar graphs represent value ranges outside of the normal reference range.

© 2003 Kronos Science, Patent Pending

CollectedDate	Patient ID	Patient Name	Accession Number
09/24/03	KCC0000003	TEST, FEMALE POSTMENOPAUSA	W2974

I- 1

FIGURE 19. Continued.

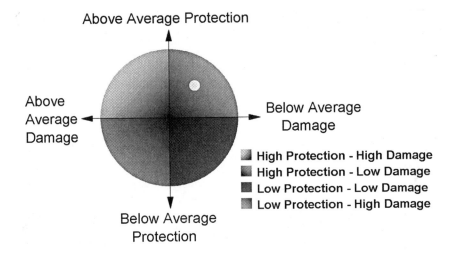

FIGURE 20. Plot of a patient's average level of antioxidant protection against their average level of oxidative damage.

SUMMARY AND CONCLUSIONS

In summary, minimization of oxidative stress appears possible through oxidative stress profiling and customized antioxidant therapy. As well, future anti-aging therapy will include upregulation of key longevity-determinant genes controlling oxidative stress and repair mechanisms through drugs and gene therapy.

REFERENCES

1. CLARKE, R. & J. ARMITAGE. 2002. Antioxidant vitamins and risk of cardiovascular disease: review of large-scale randomised trials. Cardiovasc. Drugs Ther. **16:** 411–415.
2. CUTLER, R. 1992. Genetic stability and oxidative stress: common mechanisms in aging and cancer. *In* Free Radicals and Aging. I. Emerit & B. Chance, Eds.: 31–46. Birkhauer Verlag. Basel.
3. CUTLER, R.G. 2003. Genetic stability, dysdifferentiation, and longevity determinant genes. *In* Critical Reviews of Oxidative Stress and Aging: Advances in Basic Science, Diagnostics and Intervention, Vol. 2. R.G. Cutler & H. Rodriguez, Eds.: 1136–1235. World Scientific. Singapore.
4. FINKEL, T. & N.J. HOLBROOK. 2000. Oxidants, oxidative stress and the biology of ageing. Nature **408:**239–247.
5. CUTLER, R.G. 1995. Oxidative Stress and Aging. Birkhauser Verlag. Basel.

6. AUSTAD, S. N. 1997. Why We Age: What Science is Discovering about the Body's Journey through Life. Wiley. New York.

7. HALLIWELL, B. & J. M.C. GUTTERIDGE. 1999. Free radicals in biology and medicine. Oxford University Press. New York.

8. CUTLER, R.G. 1975. Evolution of human longevity and the genetic complexity governing aging rate. Proc. Natl. Acad. Sci. USA **72:** 4664–4668.

9. CUTLER, R. 1976. Evolution of longevity in primates. J. Hum. Evol. **5:**169–202.

10. CUTLER, R.G. 1979. Evolution of longevity in ungulates and carnivores. Gerontology **25:** 69–86.

11. CUTLER, R.G. 1982. Longevity is determined by specific genes: testing the hypothesis. *In* Testing the Theories of Aging. R.A. Roth & G.S. Roth, Eds.: 25–114. CRC Press. Boca Raton, FL.

12. CUTLER, R.G. 1984. Carotenoids and retinol: their possible importance in determining longevity of primate species. Proc. Natl. Acad. Sci. USA **81:** 7627–7631.

13. CUTLER, R.G. 1984. Urate and ascorbate: their possible roles as antioxidants in determining longevity of mammalian species. Arch. Gerontol. Geriatr. **3:** 321–348.

14. CUTLER, R.G. 1985. Peroxide-producing potential of tissues: inverse correlation with longevity of mammalian species. Proc. Natl. Acad. Sci. USA **82:** 4798–4802.

15. CUTLER, R.G. 1985. Antioxidants and longevity of mammalian species. *In* Molecular Biology of Aging. A.D. Woodhead & A. Hollaender, Eds.: 15–74. Plenum Press. New York.

16. CUTLER, R. 1990. Liver cytochrome P-450 detoxification system: possible role in human aging and longevity. *In* Liver and Aging. K. Kitani, Ed.: 337–351. Elsevier. Limerick, Ireland.

17. CUTLER, R. 1991. Antioxidants and aging. Am J. Clin Nutr. **53:** 373s–379s.

18. ANISIMOV, V.N. 2003. Insulin/IGF-1 signaling pathway driving aging and cancer as a target for pharmacological intervention. Exp. Gerontol. **38:**041–1049.

19. LIN, K. *et al.* 1997. daf-16: An HNF-3/forkhead family member that can function to double the life-span of Caenorhabditis elegans. Science. **278:**1319–1322.

20. FINCH, C.E. & G. RUVKUN. 2001. The genetics of aging. Annu. Rev. Genomics Hum. Genet. **2:** 435–462.

21. LIN, Y.J., L. SEROUDE & S. BENZER. 1998. Extended life-span and stress resistance in the *Drosophila* mutant methuselah. Science **282:** 943–946.

22. KENYON, C. 2001. A conserved regulatory system for aging. Cell **105:**165–168.

23. CUTLER, R.G. 1993. Genetic and evolutionary molecular aspects of aging. Academic Press 25–58.

24. CUTLER, R.G. 1995. Oxidative stress: its potential relevance to human disease and longevity determinants. Age :91–96.

25. CUTLER, R.G. & H. RODRIGUEZ. 2003. Critical Reviews of Oxidative Stress and Aging: Advances in Basic Science, Diagnostics and Intervention. World Scientific. Singapore.

26. ARKING, R. 1998. Biology of aging: observations and principles. Sinauer Associates. Sunderland, MA.

    TROEN, B.R. 2003. The biology of aging. Mt. Sinai J. Med. **70:** 3–22.

    AARON, H.J. 2000. The Centenarian Boom. Brookings Review. **18.**

29. Garcia-Arumi, E. *et al.* 1998. Effect of oxidative stress on lymphocytes from elderly subjects. Clin. Sci. (Lond.). **94:** 447–452.
30. Herskind, A.M. *et al.* 1996. The heritability of human longevity: a population-based study of 2872 Danish twin pairs born 1870-1900. Hum. Genet. **97:** 319–323.
31. Larkin, M. 1999. Centenarians point the way to healthy ageing. Lancet. **353:** 1074.
32. Longo, V.D. & C.E. Finch. 2003. Evolutionary medicine: from dwarf model systems to healthy centenarians? Science **299:** 1342–1346.
33. Perls, T.T. *et al.* 1998. Siblings of centenarians live longer. Lancet **351:** 1560.
34. Perls, T.T. *et al.* 2002. Life-long sustained mortality advantage of siblings of centenarians. Proc. Natl. Acad. Sci. USA **99:** 8442–8447.
35. Perls, T. & A. Puca. 2002. The genetics of aging–implications for pharmaco-genomics. Pharmacogenomics **3:** 469–484.
36. Perls, T. 2001. Genetic and phenotypic markers among centenarians. J. Gerontol. A Biol. Sci. Med. Sci. **56:** M67–70.
37. Perls, T, *et al.* 2000. Exceptional familial clustering for extreme longevity in humans. J. Am. Geriatr. Soc. **48:** 1483–1485.
38. Plaskin, G. 2001. Secrets of the centenarians. Family Circle **2:** 36.
39. Schachter, F. 1998. Causes, effects, and constraints in the genetics of human longevity. Am. J. Hum. Genet. **62:** 1008–1014.
40. Tanaka, M. *et al.* 2000. Mitochondrial genotype associated with longevity and its inhibitory effect on mutagenesis. Mech. Ageing Dev. **116:** 65–76.
41. van Bockxmeer, F.M. 1994. ApoE and ACE genes: impact on human longevity. Nat. Genet. **6:** 4–5.
42. Yashin, A.I. *et al.* 2000. Genes and longevity: lessons from studies of centenarians. J. Gerontol. A Biol. Sci. Med. Sci. **55:** B319–328.
43. Zhang, J. *et al.* 2003. Strikingly higher frequency in centenarians and twins of mtDNA mutation causing remodeling of replication origin in leukocytes. Proc. Natl. Acad. Sci. USA. **100:** 1116–1121.
44. Holliday, R. 1995. Understanding Ageing. Cambridge University Press. New York.
45. Cutler, R.G. 1973. Redundancy of information content in the genome of mammalian species as a protective mechanism determining aging rate. Mech. Ageing Dev. **2:** 381–408.
46. Cutler, R.G. 1972. Transcription of reiterated DNA sequence classes throughout the life-span of the mouse. *In* Advances in Gerontological Research, Vol. 4. B.S. Strehler, Ed.: 220–340. Academic Press. New York.
47. Cutler, R.G. 1976. Nature of aging and life maintenance processes. *In* Interdisciplinary Topics in Gerontology, Vol. 9. R.G. Cutler, Ed.: 83–133. S. Karger. Basel.
48. Austad, S.N. 1997. Comparative aging and life histories in mammals. Exp. Gerontol. **32:** 23–38.
49. Brommer, J.E. 2000. The evolution of fitness in life-history theory. Biol. Rev. Camb. Philos. Soc. **75:** 377–404.
50. Kirkwood, T.B. 1992. Comparative life spans of species: why do species have the life spans they do? Am. J. Clin. Nutr. **55:** 1191S–1195S.
51. Kapahi, P., M.E. Boulton & T.B. Kirkwood. 1999. Positive correlation between mammalian life span and cellular resistance to stress. Free Radic. Biol. Med. **26:**495–500.

52. 2002. Time, cells, and Strehler. Special section in memory of Bernard L. Strehler. Mech. Ageing Dev. 123: 819–993.

53. RIGGS, J.E. & R.J. MILLECCHIA. 1992. Using the Gompertz-Strehler model of aging and mortality to explain mortality trends in industrialized countries. Mech Ageing Dev. **65**:217–228.

54. ARANTES-OLIVEIRA, N., J.R. BERMAN & C. KENYON. 2003. Healthy animals with extreme longevity. Science **302:**611.

55. FINCH, C.E. 1990. Longevity, senescence, and the genome. University of Chicago Press. Chicago.

56. CUTLER, R.G. 1972. Transcription of reiterated DNA sequence classes throughout the life-span of the mouse. Adv. Gerontological. Res. **4:**219–321.

57. ARANTES-OLIVEIRA, N., *et al.* 2002. Regulation of life-span by germ-line stem cells in *Caenorhabditis elegans*. Science **295:**502–505.

58. BARBIERI, M. *et al.* 2003. Insulin/IGF-I-signaling pathway: an evolutionarily conserved mechanism of longevity from yeast to humans. Am. J. Physiol. Endocrinol. Metab. **285:**E1064–1071.

59. KIRKWOOD, T.B. 2003. Genes that shape the course of ageing. Trends Endocrinol. Metab. **14:**345–347.

60. INTERNATIONAL LONGEVITY CENTER-USA. n.d. Longevity Genes from Primative Organisms to Humans. Report of workshop held under the auspices of the American Federation for Aging Research and the Glenn Foundation for Medical Research.

61. KIRKWOOD, T.B. & M.R. ROSE. 1991. Evolution of senescence: late survival sacrificed for reproduction. Philos. Trans. R. Soc. Lond. B Biol. Sci. **332:** 15–24.

62. ROSE, M.R. 1991. Evolutionary Biology of Aging. Oxford University Press. New York.

63. WALLACE, D.C. 1967. The inevitability of growing old. J. Chronic Dis. **20:** 475–486.

64. WALLACE, D.C. 1975. A theory of the cause of aging. Med. J. Aust. **1:** 829–831.

65. WILLIAMS, P.D. & T. DAY. 2003. Antagonistic pleiotropy, mortality source interactions, and the evolutionary theory of senescence. Evolution Int. J. Org. Evol. **57:** 1478–1488.

66. HAMILTON, W.D. 1966. The moulding of senescence by natural selection. J. Theor. Biol. **12:** 12–45.

67. CHARLESWORTH, B. 2000. Fisher, Medawar, Hamilton and the evolution of aging. Genetics **156:** 927–931.

68. CUTLER, R. 1976. Nature of Aging and Life Maintenance Processes. Interdisc. Topics Gerontol. **9:** 83–133.

69. BLIZNAKOV, E.G. 1999. Cardiovascular diseases, oxidative stress and antioxidants: the decisive role of coenzyme Q10. Cardiovasc. Res. **43:** 248–249.

70. FORSBERG, L., U. DE FAIRE & R. MORGENSTERN. 2001. Oxidative stress, human genetic variation, and disease. Arch. Biochem. Biophys. **389:** 84–93.

71. ENGELHARDT, J.F., C.K. SEN & L. OBERLEY. 2001. Redox-modulating gene therapies for human diseases. Antioxid. Redox Signal. **3:** 341–346.

72. KISHIMOTO, C., *et al.* 2001. Serum thioredoxin (TRX) levels in patients with heart failure. Jpn. Circ. J. **65:** 491–494.

73. SIEMS, W., *et al.* 2003. Carotenoid cleavage products modify respiratory burst and induce apoptosis of human neutrophils. Biochim. Biophys. Acta **1639:** 27–33.

74. WAGNER, K.H. & I. ELMADFA. 2003. Biological relevance of terpenoids: overview focusing on mono-, di- and tetraterpenes. Ann. Nutr. Metab. **47:** 95–106.
75. BECKMAN, K.B. & B.N. AMES. 1998. The free radical theory of aging matures. Physiol. Rev. **78:** 547–581.
76. WAKABAYASHI, N., *et al.* 2004. Protection against electrophile and oxidant stress by induction of the phase 2 response: fate of cysteines of the Keap1 sensor modified by inducers. Proc. Natl. Acad. Sci. USA **101:** 2040–2045.
77. GAO, X. & P. TALALAY. 2004. Induction of phase 2 genes by sulforaphane protects retinal pigment epithelial cells against photooxidative damage. Proc. Natl. Acad. Sci. USA **101:** 10446–10451.
78. CUTLER, R.G. 1992. Genetic stability and oxidative stress: common mechanisms in aging and cancer. Exs. **62:** 31–46.
79. STOHS, S.J. 1995. The role of free radicals in toxicity and disease. J. Basic Clin. Physiol. Pharmacol. **6:** 205–228.
80. WEI, Y.H. 1998. Oxidative stress and mitochondrial DNA mutations in human aging. Proc. Soc. Exp. Biol. Med. **217:** 53–63.
81. MUNCH, G. *et al.* 1997. Advanced glycation endproducts in ageing and Alzheimer's disease. Brain Res. Brain Res .Rev. **23:** 134–143.
82. THORPE, S.R. & J.W. BAYNES. 1996. Role of the Maillard reaction in diabetes mellitus and diseases of aging. Drugs Aging. **9:** 69–77.
83. BASTIANETTO, S. *et al.* 1999. Dehydroepiandrosterone (DHEA) protects hippo campal cells from oxidative stress-induced damage. Brain Res. Mol. Brain Res. **66:** 35–41.
84. COOKSON, M.R. & P.J. SHAW. 1999. Oxidative stress and motor neurone disease. Brain Pathol. **9:** 165–186.
85. TOLMASOFF, J.M., T. ONO & R.G. CUTLER. 1980. Superoxide dismutase: correlation with life-span and specific metabolic rate in primate species. Proc. Natl. Acad. Sci USA **77:** 2777–2781.
86. ONO, T. & S. OKADA. 1984. Unique increase of superoxide dismutase level in brains of long living mammals. Exp. Gerontol. **19:** 349–354.
87. SOHAL, R.S., B.H. SOHAL & W.C. ORR. 1995. Mitochondrial superoxide and hydrogen peroxide generation, protein oxidative damage, and longevity in different species of flies. Free Radic. Biol. Med. **19:** 499–504.
88. BARJA, G., *et al.* 1994. A decrease of free radical production near critical targets as a cause of maximum longevity in animals. Comp. Biochem. Physiol. Biochem. Mol. Biol. **108:** 501–512.
89. BARJA, G., *et al.* 1994. Low mitochondrial free radical production per unit O_2 consumption can explain the simultaneous presence of high longevity and high aerobic metabolic rate in birds. Free Radic. Res. **21:** 317–327.
90. BARJA, G. 1999. Mitochondrial oxygen radical generation and leak: sites of production in states 4 and 3, organ specificity, and relation to aging and longevity. J. Bioenerg. Biomembr. **31:** 347–366.
91. BARJA, G. 2000. The flux of free radical attack through mitochondrial DNA is related to aging rate. Aging (Milan) **12:** 342–355.
92. BARJA, G. 2002. Rate of generation of oxidative stress-related damage and animal longevity. Free Radic. Biol. Med. **33:** 1167–1172.
93. CUTLER, R.G. 1985. Urate and ascorbate: their possible role as antioxidants in determining longevity of mammalian species. Arch. Gerontol. Geriatrics. **3:** 321–348.

94. CAO, G., H.M. ALESSIO & R.G. CUTLER. 1993. Oxygen-radical absorbance capacity assay for antioxidants. Free Radic. Biol. Med. **14:** 303–311.

95. PEREZ-CAMPO, R. *et al.* 1998. The rate of free radical production as a determinant of the rate of aging: evidence from the comparative approach. J. Comp. Physiol. [B]. **168:** 149–58.

96. PEREZ-CAMPO, R. *et al.* 1994. Longevity and antioxidant enzymes, non-enzymatic antioxidants and oxidative stress in the vertebrate lung: a comparative study. J. Comp. Physiol. [B]. **163:** 682–689.

97. PAMPLONA, R., G. BARJA & M. PORTERO-OTIN. 2002. Membrane fatty acid unsaturation, protection against oxidative stress, and maximum life span: a homeoviscous-longevity adaptation? Ann. N.Y. Acad. Sci. **959:** 475–490.

98. PEREZ-CAMPO, R. *et al.* 1993. A comparative study of free radicals in vertebrates–I. Antioxidant enzymes. Comp. Biochem. Physiol. B. **105:** 749–755.

99. PAMPLONA, R. *et al.* 2000. Low fatty acid unsaturation: a mechanism for lowered lipoperoxidative modification of tissue proteins in mammalian species with long life spans. J. Gerontol. A Biol. Sci. Med. Sci. **55:** B286–291.

100. PAMPLONA, R. *et al.* 2000. Double bond content of phospholipids and lipid peroxidation negatively correlate with maximum longevity in the heart of mammals. Mech. Ageing Dev. **112:** 169–183.

101. PAMPLONA, R. *et al.* 1999. Heart fatty acid unsaturation and lipid peroxidation, and aging rate, are lower in the canary and the parakeet than in the mouse. Aging (Milano). **11:** 44–49.

102. PAMPLONA, R. *et al.* 1999. A low degree of fatty acid unsaturation leads to lower lipid peroxidation and lipoxidation-derived protein modification in heart mitochondria of the longevous pigeon than in the short-lived rat. Mech. Ageing Dev. **106:** 283–296.

103. PAMPLONA, R. *et al.* 1996. Low fatty acid unsaturation protects against lipid peroxidation in liver mitochondria from long-lived species: the pigeon and human case. Mech. Ageing Dev. **86:** 53–66.

104. HERRERO, A. *et al.* 2001. Effect of the degree of fatty acid unsaturation of rat heart mitochondria on their rates of H2O2 production and lipid and protein oxidative damage. Mech. Ageing Dev. **122:** 427–443.

105. ADELMAN, R., R.L. SAUL & B.N. AMES. 1988. Oxidative damage to DNA: relation to species metabolic rate and life span. Proc. Natl. Acad. Sci. USA **85:** 2706–2708.

106. PARK, J.W., K.C. CUNDY & B.N. AMES. 1989. Detection of DNA adducts by high-performance liquid chromatography with electrochemical detection. Carcinogenesis **10:** 827–832.

107. HELBOCK, H.J., K.B. BECKMAN & B.N. AMES. 1999. 8-Hydroxydeoxyguanosine and 8-hydroxyguanine as biomarkers of oxidative DNA damage. Methods Enzymol. **300:** 156–166.

108. SHIGENAGA, M.K., C.J. GIMENO & B.N. AMES. 1989. Urinary 8-hydroxy-2'-deoxyguanosine as a biological marker of in vivo oxidative DNA damage. Proc. Natl. Acad. Sci. USA **86:** 9697–9701.

109. CATHCART, R. *et al.* 1984. Thymine glycol and thymidine glycol in human and rat urine: a possible assay for oxidative DNA damage. Proc. Natl. Acad. Sci. USA **81:**5633–5637.

110. HIROTA, K., *et al.* 2002. Thioredoxin superfamily and thioredoxin-inducing agents. Ann. N.Y. Acad. Sci. **957:** 189–199.

111. MITSUI, A. *et al.* 2002. Overexpression of human thioredoxin in transgenic mice controls oxidative stress and life span. Antioxid. Redox Signal. **4:** 693–696.
112. NAKAMURA, H., A. MITSUI & J. YODOI. 2002. Thioredoxin overexpression in transgenic mice. Methods Enzymol. **347:** 436–440.
113. SHIOJI, K., *et al.* 2002. Overexpression of thioredoxin-1 in transgenic mice attenuates adriamycin-induced cardiotoxicity. Circulation **106:** 1403–1409.
114. TAKAGI, Y., *et al.* 1999. Overexpression of thioredoxin in transgenic mice attenuates focal ischemic brain damage. Proc. Natl. Acad. Sci. USA. **96:** 4131–4136.
115. YOSHIDA, T. *et al.* 2003. The role of thioredoxin in the aging process: involvement of oxidative stress. Antioxid. Redox Signal. **5:** 563–570.
116. MARTIN, G.M. & L.A. LOEB. 2004. Ageing: mice and mitochondria. Nature **429:** 357–359.
117. ORSINI, F., *et al.* 2004. The life span determinant p66Shc localizes to mitochondria where it associates with mitochondrial heat shock protein 70 and regulates trans-membrane potential. J. Biol. Chem. **279:** 25689–25695.
118. PACINI, S. *et al.* 2004. p66SHC promotes apoptosis and antagonizes mitogenic signaling in T cells. Mol. Cell Biol. **24:** 1747–1757.
119. NAPOLI, C. *et al.* 2003. Deletion of the p66Shc longevity gene reduces systemic and tissue oxidative stress, vascular cell apoptosis, and early atherogenesis in mice fed a high-fat diet. Proc. Natl. Acad. Sci. USA **100:** 2112–2116.
120. VENTURA, A. *et al.* 2002. The p66Shc longevity gene is silenced through epigenetic modifications of an alternative promoter. J. Biol. Chem. **277:** 22370–22376.
121. ONO, T. *et al.* 1985. Dysdifferentiative nature of aging: age-dependent expression of MuLV and globin genes in thymus, liver and brain in the AKR mouse strain. Gerontology **31:** 362–372.
122. CUTLER, R.G. 1982. The dysdifferentiative hypothesis of mammalian aging and longevity. *In* The Aging Brain: Cellular and Molecular Mechanisms of Aging in the Nervous System. E. Giacobini *et al.* Eds.: 1–19. Raven Press. New York.
123. DEAN, R.G., S.H. SOCHER & R.G. CUTLER. 1985. Dysdifferentiative nature of aging: age-dependent expression of mouse mammary tumor virus and casein genes in brain and liver tissues of the C57BL/6J mouse strain. Arch. Gerontol. Geriatr. **4:** 43–51.
124. KATOR, K. *et al.* 1985. Dysdifferentiative nature of aging: passage number dependency of globin gene expression in normal human diploid cells grown in tissue culture. Gerontology **31:** 355–361.
125. ZS-NAGY, I., R.G. CUTLER & I. SEMSEI. 1988. Dysdifferentiation hypothesis of aging and cancer: a comparison with the membrane hypothesis of aging. Ann. N.Y. Acad. Sci. **521:** 215–225.
126. CUTLER, R.G. & I. SEMSEI. 1989. Development, cancer and aging: possible common mechanisms of action and regulation. J. Gerontol. **44:** 25–34.
127. CUTLER, R.G. 1991. Recent progress in testing the longevity determinant and dysdifferentiation hypotheses of aging. Arch. Gerontol. Geriatr. **12:** 75–98.
128. GAUBATZ, J.W., B. ARCEMENT & R.G. CUTLER. 1991. Gene expression of an endogenous retrovirus-like element during murine development and aging. Mech. Ageing Dev. **57:** 71–85.
129. BAFITIS, H. & F. SARGENT, 2ND. 1977. Human psychological adaptability through the life sequence. J. Gerontol. 32: 402–410.

Oxidative Stress Profiling

Part II. Theory, Technology, and Practice

RICHARD G. CUTLER, JOHN PLUMMER, KAJAL CHOWDHURY, AND CHRISTOPHER HEWARD

Kronos Science Laboratories, Phoenix, Arizona 85016, USA

ABSTRACT: Many of the most serious human diseases have a strong association with the steady-state level of oxidative damage in tissues. On an individual level this damage is defined as the patient's *oxidative stress status* (OSS). OSS is associated with many of the major age-related diseases such as cancer, heart disease, diabetes, and Alzheimer's disease, as well as with the aging process itself. In general, the greater the OSS of the individual, the higher the risk for disease development. To further understand the role that OSS has as a causative or an associated factor for these diseases, and to develop more effective personalized therapy to minimize OSS, requires a reliable means to measure the many different components contributing to an individual's OSS. This procedure is called *oxidative stress profiling* (OSP) and represents a new strategy to simultaneously assess an individual's OSS as well as to identify key physiological parameters, such as the hormone, lipid, antioxidant, or iron profile, that may be responsible for that individual's OSS. The OSP strategy provides physicians with information that enable them to make a more accurate diagnosis of the patient's condition and to recommend specific types of therapy based on better scientific data. Follow-up studies of the patient would then be conducted using these same tests until the OSS of the patient has been minimized. The OSP strategy is particularly well suited for a personalized health optimization program. The procedure is based on measuring both the steady-state levels of oxidative damage in nucleic acids, proteins, and lipids and the protective and defense processes of these components using blood, urine, and breath samples. Testing individuals before and after a controlled amount of exercise (70% VO_2) may also help to obtain greater sensitivity and reproducibility. Evaluation of test results to obtain an integrated calculated OSS result for a patient represents a major challenge. One approach is to present the test results on a percentile bases, allowing results of different tests to be integrated into one or a few parameters, such as an oxidative stress and an antioxidant index. This article presents a general overview and rationale of the concept of the oxidative stress profile, tests to be used, and examples of how it may be applied.

Address for correspondence: Dr. Richard Cutler, Kronos Science Laboratories, Inc., 2222 East Highland Avenue, Suite 220, Phoenix, AZ 85016. Voice: 602-778-7488; fax: 602-667-5623
richard.cutler@kronoslaboratory.com

Ann. N.Y. Acad. Sci. 1055: 136–158 (2005). © 2005 New York Academy of Sciences.
doi: 10.1196/annals.1323.031

KEYWORDS: free radicals; oxidative stress profile; longevity; aging; reactive oxygen species; cellular aging

INTRODUCTION

Free Radical Biology and Chemistry

What are free radicals, ROS and RNS? Reactive oxygen species (ROS) and reactive nitrogen species (RNS) are free radical products produced in all aerobic organisms. These free radical species can in principle react and/or alter or destroy most all cellular constituents.[1–3]

Why do they exist? The presence of these free radicals in biological systems represents an evolutionary pleiotropic effect. These are the beneficial effects free radicals have to the organism that outweigh their more toxic effects. For example, in the process of producing required energy in mitochondria (ATP), toxic ROS/RNS are also produced through the oxygen's being utilized.[4–7]

All organisms represent a history of evolutionary trade-offs. These processes played an important central role in molding the many different and interacting processes making up all living organisms.[8–15] For example, take any given metabolic pathway and you can identify both advantages and disadvantages in its design, the biochemical and enzyme components involved, and the end product. Nothing is ever perfect in biology, despite beliefs to the contrary, and there always appear to be pleiotropic effects. Such is the case for the utilization of oxygen in the production of energy in aerobic organisms. The trade-off is efficient energy production (ATP) against the toxic side effects of the ROS and RNS created as a pleiotropic side effect of this process. Later, new strategies evolved, taking advantage of some of these toxic byproducts, as in immune defense mechanisms, secondary messengers, and in redox signaling.

Co-evolution of aging and anti-aging (longevity) processes. A similar pleiotropic-effect explanation has been used to explain the co-evolution of aging and anti-aging processes.[16–18] Aging of the organism is proposed to be the resulting byproduct of normal processes essential for maintaining life. That is, aging did not evolve as an evolutionary selected process. Instead, aging is the result of the natural instability of necessary biological materials and toxic byproducts of essential reactions that evolved for other purposes. Thus, it is nonsense to speak of the evolution of aging. On the other hand, anti-aging or longevity did evolve when the advantage of longer life outweighed the disadvantage of the pleiotropic anti-aging processes. Some of the mechanisms involved in the evolution of anti-aging or longevity processes have been proposed to include increased resistance, protection, and repair processes against the cellular damage produced by the endogenous generation of free radicals.

The Sources of ROS/RNS Production in Eukaryotic Cells

In eukaryotic cells the major source of ROS/RNS is the mitochondrion.[4,19] Mitochondria are the natural byproducts of the oxidative phosphorylation reaction producing energy in the form of ATP from oxygen. Another important source is the production of ROS/RNS from macrophage cells during the oxygen burst process.[20] Here the ROS/RNS act to destroy foreign organisms such as bacteria. However, continued low-grade chronic infection and other stimulants of this source of reactive species can result in a low-grade chronic state of inflammation, contributing to many of the age-related related diseases.[21–23]

How do ROS/RNS Cause Cellular and Organism Dysfunction?

Destruction of essential cellular and structural components. It is clear many of the endogenously produced free radicals have sufficient energy to destroy any molecule or structure within a cell, leading to disease or death of the organism. A simple view of how ROS/RNS reduce cell function is their destruction of cellular components so that proper function is no longer possible. Therefore, are all components of a cell of equal importance as sensitive targets, or are there particular targets that, when damaged, produce the most serious and far-reaching dysfunctional effects?

The answer to this question has usually been nuclear DNA or mitochondrial DNA as being the most important target. In fact, a popular hypothesis is that because free radicals are well known to be mutagenic, their most serious effect is related to their mutagenic properties.[24] Another hypothesis is that, with time, there is an accumulation of non-repairable damage throughout the entire cell. This steady accumulation of damage results in a decrease in functional capacity of most physiological processes. A wear-and-tear process occurs gradually, decreasing the amount of normally available cellular components. This results in an increasing cascade of cellular/organism dysfunction on many levels.

How does ROS/RNS Cause Aging?

The wear-and-tear oxidative stress hypothesis of aging. A similar hypothesis, generally known as the free radical theory of aging, has been proposed describing how free radicals can cause aging.[24–28] The basic idea is that cells in old organisms become so loaded with free radical–mediated damage that the cell/tissues can no longer carry out a normal minimum level of functions.[29,30] This leads to a steady decrease in physiological functional capacity of cells, tissues, and then, the whole organism. On the basis of this free radical theory of aging, it has recently been seriously proposed that the removal or cleaning up of the free damaged components existing in an old animal would result in its rejuvenation or return to youthful condition.[31]

The dysdifferentiation hypothesis of aging. Many years ago, I (R.G.C.) presented another hypothesis of how free radicals cause aging.[16,32–34] It was proposed that the most sensitive target of free radicals, which result in the most serious consequences when occurring at low normal dosage levels, are those processes within a cell that are involved in the control and maintenance of the proper differentiated state of the cell. I have also proposed that free radicals produce this dysdifferentiation process largely through epigenetic instead of mutational mechanisms.[33,35–37] For example, free radical modification of chromatin protein structure, regulatory proteins, or transcription factors in the cytoplasm or nucleus could perturb proper transcription profiles, resulting in a stable but less efficient and improper alteration in the differentiated state of a cell.

This concept has been described as the *dysdifferentiation hypothesis of aging*.[33,38,39] Its unique feature is that a little damage can be greatly amplified in terms of having small but long-term serious effects. This dysdifferentiation hypothesis of aging has the interesting feature of suggesting that aging is more like the reverse of the very epigenetically mediated differentiation and developmental processes that created the organism in the first place. Another interesting feature of this hypothesis is that recent evidence now supports an important role of epigenetic processes operating in the etiology of cancer as well as mutational events. Thus, the well known age-related increase in cancer may simply represent a special case of dysdifferentiation (specific genes are effected as oncogenes) of the general aging process where genes controlling differentiation are mostly affected.

In this dysdifferentiation hypothesis of aging, the mechanism controlling aging rate, life span, and the general maintenance of function and general health, are those processes controlling the stability of the proper differentiated state of cells. The connection to oxidative stress is that oxidative stress acts to perturb differentiation largely through epigenetic mechanisms. Although little is known about the process stabilizing differentiation, one mechanism involves those processes that control the oxidative stress state of a cell or its oxidative/reductive status

The stem cell epigenetic dysdifferentiation hypothesis of aging. It appears now that the primary mechanism of general maintenance of all tissues in an organism is through a specific set of stem cells specific for each tissue type.[40–44] However, these stem cells gradually lose their special state of differentiation, largely through epigenetic drift rather than mutational mechanisms, and as a result the tissues that had depended on their renewal become increasingly defective through an impaired chromatin and tissue remodeling process.[45–48] It was suggested (by R.G.C.) that the age-dependent epigenetic improper alterations of the stem cells are enhanced by free radical mechanisms (ROS/RNS) and that, in turn, the rate of dysdifferentiation of the stem cells would in part be controlled by processes controlling the oxidative stress status of those stem cells.

Thus, in this model, the aging process of an organism is the result of epigenetic mechanisms operating at the levels of the stem cell tissue renewal system that produce defective remodeled or "aged" tissue. In turn, life span of a species would be dependent upon the degree to which stem cells can maintain their proper differentiation state; this would in part be controlled by the oxidative stress status of the cells. It would therefore be predicted that human stem cells can maintain their proper state of differentiation for more generations (and more time) than those of shorter-lived primates or mammalian species. Certain model organisms, as in some invertebrates, where most tissues are postmitotic in nature and not dependent on stem cell renewal maintenance (nematode and *Drosophila*), would fail to represent the situation existing in mammalian organisms. Thus, if all tissues of an organism are maintained through renewal processes coming from a stem cell population, it follows that perhaps the most important target to protect against free radical–mediated dysdifferentiation are these stem cells.

The concept of longevity-determinant genes. A number of years ago, it was also proposed that in spite of the vast complexity of aging processes, relative simple processes exist that act to control the rate of aging.[16,17,39,49] These processes are controlled by a speciate class of genes called longevity-determinant genes (LDGs). One class of LDGs would then include those key genes that control the oxidative stress status of a cell, which would be particularly important for the stem cell population.

Free radicals are also involved in a process called glycosylation, which represents another beautiful example of the pleiotropic nature of aging processes.[50–54] Here, the many advantages of certain class of sugar molecules (such as glucose) have for cell function, particularly in energy pathways, are important in cell evolution. Yet, these same molecules are inherently unstable, particularly in the presence of free radicals resulting in the formation of toxic compounds, for example less functional collagen cross-linked tissues. Hyperglycemic conditions are also found to increase the free radial leakage from mitochondria.

These glycosylation reactions appear to be most important as an explanation of the disease processes associated with diabetes type II, where reduction of free radiated–mediated cellular damage is a promising means of therapy. Indeed, there are many examples like this in which free radicals act to amplify inherent instabilities in an organism.

In summary, there is not yet sufficient information as to what mechanism free radicals use to alter proper cell function. There is, however, compelling information indicating that disease, age-related disease, and aging rate are all associated with the general intensity of oxidative stress occurring within a cell.[38] Clearly, for oxidative stress profiling to work most efficiently and economically, it is critical to know the most sensitive targets to oxidation, those resulting in the greatest far-reaching biological dysfunctional effects. Thus, measurement of oxidation of critical components in chromatin, as in nucleosomes assessing degree of epigenetic alteration, may be better than measuring an oxidized serum component. It also follows that biomarkers of aging may be more successful if they measure alterations more closely associated with the origin of the aging process itself, such as the degree of dysdifferentiation occurring within specific cells of an organism, rather than a decrease in physiological functions of an organ system.

What are the Processes That Have Evolved to Reduce the Destructive Effects of ROS/RNS?

The endogenous generation of highly reactive free radicals within a cell is so high that it is clear that essential protection of a cell is necessary to avoid immediate destruction and death. A number of such protective/defense processes have been identified.[55–68]

First line of defense: reduce endogenous production of free radicals. One of the first lines of protection is to reduce the rate of free radicals produced per amount of oxygen utilized in all cells. This could occur by reducing free radical leakage from mitochondria (perhaps through mitochondria uncoupling proteins) or from cells involved in producing chronic inflammation reactions. Therefore, cells from long-lived organisms, such as humans, might be expected to produce fewer free radical molecules leaking from the mitochondria (amount of oxygen used per amount of ATP molecule produced) as compared to mitochondria from cells of a chimpanzee, which has half the life span. There is some evidence that mitochondria are indeed more efficient in longer-lived organisms.

Second line of defense: Reduce specific metabolic rate (SMR). A related line of defense is to simply decrease metabolic rate. This can be done with an accompanied advantage of lowering environmental hazards of an animal by simply becoming larger. Larger animals require less energy expenditure to maintain a given body temperature than do smaller animals, simply because of a lesser ratio of surface area to total body mass. Support for this concept is the excellent correlation of life span with body size of most mammalian species. Humans are, however, an exception to this rule, considering their long life span and relative small body size. This can be readily explained by human tissues' having higher levels of antioxidant protection.

Third line of defense: Increase resistance of key targets to oxidative stress damage. Another mechanism to increase defense against free radicals is for an organism to increase the resistance of key components of a cell structure to oxidative damage. A good example here is the inverse relationship of the peroxidizability of the membrane and other cellular components of tissues to a species' life span. This has been explained by the decrease in composition of peroxidizable fatty acid molecules in cellular membranes, such as the un-saturated fatty acids.

Fourth line of defense: Increase protection against free radicals by remov-ing them by antioxidants. This line of defense comes from a class of mole-cules called antioxidants. Antioxidants include enzymes that catalytically remove free radicals (as superoxide dismutase removes the superoxide radi-cal) and molecules that sacrificially react with free radicals, thus removing the free radical, but also, at the same time, becoming a less toxic free radical itself (such as alpha tocopherol). These antioxidants are synthesized endoge-nously, as is uric acid,, but are also an important part of the diet as the caro-tenoids or tocopherols. There is much evidence that longer-lived species do indeed have higher levels of the same antioxidants in their tissues and blood than do shorter-lived species.

Fifth line of defense: Repair, turnover, or remodeling processes. Perhaps the most fundamental mechanism protecting cells and organisms from the toxic accumulative effects of free radical damage is the renewal or remodel-ing processes. Examples include cell division, DNA replication, and general tissue renewal and remodeling processes. All of these processes result in re-moval of damaged components. However, the efficiency is greatly increased if the rate of removable components is greater for cell/molecules that are ab-normal or have been oxidized or damaged by free radicals. There is experi-mental support for this prediction, particularly for the action of the proteosome. However, general rate of tissue turnover and renewal is actually inversely related to the life span of different species. Selection for removal of oxidized cellular components must operate for this line of defense to be effective.

Sixth line of defense: Repair processes for nucleic acid, protein, and lipid components of a cell. Finally, there is the important class of repair processes that exists for the nucleic acids, proteins, and lipids. These repair processes specifically recognize oxidative damage and they repair that damage, reju-venating the function for the molecule. There is some evidence that such re-pair processes, as for DNA excision repair, are more active in longer-lived organisms.

WHAT IS MEANT BY OXIDATIVE STRESS AND OXIDATIVE STRESS STATUS?

The concepts of what process are involved in producing oxidative damage. and those that act in protecting and repairing oxidative damage, lead naturally to the concept of oxidative stress and oxidative stress status.[69–76] The most accepted definition as to what is meant by oxidative stress is based on the concept that there is a normal rate of production of free radicals for a given average oxygen consumption rate. A majority of the free radicals produced are removed by antioxidants. Only a few are eventually able to reach a target and produce damage.

Now most of this damage is removed by repair or selective degradation turnover processes. Thus, we have a situation of establishing a state of equilibrium where rate of input of damage will equal the rate of output of damage, assuming that all damage is eventually repaired. It is this unrepaired damage that is predicted to increase with age. This steady-state rate of damage-in and damage-out defines the "dwell time" or average length of time the damage remains in the structure or cell before it is repaired or removed. Longer dwell times of a damaged component are likely to be more dangerous to a cell than the dwell time of short-lived damaged components. Short-lived animals, such as mice, have a very high rate of damage-in and damage-out as compared to longer-living species such as humans. In the case of the mouse, the steady-state level of oxidative damage or its oxidative stress status is much higher than in the human, even though all damage may be repaired in both mouse and human.

The concept of oxidative stress was originally defined by Dr. Helmet Sies as representing a condition where the level of oxidatively mediated damage was above what is considered normal for the cell or organism.[77–82] Thus, it represents an abnormal state that exists when a cell is considered out of balance in the in/output ratio leading to the situation where the input of damage exceeds the level of output or repair. This definition works well for some disease conditions, that is, if oxidative stress is higher than normal, only then will the disease develop.

However, the Sies definition of oxidative stress has serious disadvantages when dealing with conditions where there is not an excessof or out-of-balance number of free radicals, yet the organism nevertheless suffers a degeneration of health because of it. The classic example for this case is the normal processes of aging. To solve this problem, *we have used the term oxidative stress to define the absolute level of oxidative stress, not when free radical flux is above the normal level.*[36,83] Using this new definition of oxidative stress, zero oxidative stress occurs only when zero oxidative damage exists. Thus, oxidative stress exists by this new definition under all conditions, including the steady-state balanced condition.

We have used this definition for normal individuals because normal people age. Therefore, if free radical damage is involved as a causative factor in aging, then normal levels of damage are indeed harmful. Thus, we have proposed that rate of aging or the probability that oxidative damage leads to some type of dysfunction, is proportional to the steady-state level of oxidative damage in the cell. We have called this the oxidative stress status of the cell.

This new definition of oxidative stress is, of course, most useful for normal processes where oxidative damage still has a consequence. Aging represents a key example, but if it is proven that oxidative damage does not significantly contribute to the normal aging process, then this definition would be of less value. The Sies definition could mislead people into thinking that normal levels of oxidative stress are without any consequence or that oxidative stress is nonexistent when it is defined to be zero. Thus, throughout this paper, we will not use the Sies definition of oxidative stress. With this in mind, *oxidative stress status represents the steady-state level of oxidative damage in a given cell tissue or organism where any oxidatively mediated damage represents a stress on the structure or cell that would be better off without it.* It is also important to note that this is a linear model where oxidative damage is related to the probability of dysfunction. A parallel model would be where oxidative damage is not causatively related to disease in all cases.

This now brings up the problem of how to define more analytically the oxidative stress of a cell, tissue or organism, since it is very difficult at this time to measure all the different types of steady-state damage occurring. So, in practice we assume that the oxidative damage being measured represents only a fraction of the total oxidative damage present and clearly not the full level of oxidative damage present. It is also assumed, but not proven, that measurement of oxidative damage components in serum, urine or breath samples generally represents the condition for the whole organism.

The Effects of Oxidative Stress on Health and Aging

Supporting evidence of the potential importance of oxidative stress to human health is that more than 250 different human diseases have now been associated with oxidative stress. In addition, there have been more than 37,000 papers published in the field of oxidative stress, of which more than 7000 deal with oxidative stress and disease and 3000 with oxidative stress and aging. The yearly rate of new papers published on the topic of oxidative stress markers has increased exponentially from only 8 in 1990, 356 in 2000, and 608 in 2004. In this study, the NLM Gateway web site was used.

OXIDATIVE STRESS MARKERS IN BASIC RESEARCH

In 2004, more than 600 scientific papers were reported under the general topic of oxidative stress markers. In these papers, there was a large range of markers used to access both oxidative damage to nucleic acids, proteins and lipids, and antioxidants and antioxidant status. Most importantly, essentially all the papers were able to arrive at what they feel is a sound conclusion in their studies using these oxidative stress markers. No one reported that their accuracy or precision was insufficient or biovariation too great for the assays used to prevent any meaningful or sound conclusion to be drawn.[84–90]

DISEASES ASSOCIATED WITH OXIDATIVE STRESS

Many different human diseases and dysfunctions have now been identified to be associated with oxidative stress.[55,91] However, it should be clear that this association with oxidative stress does not have a cause-and-effect relationship. In most cases the association is secondary or beyond rather than primary. Below is only a small outline of these diseases to give the reader an idea of the wide range of human diseases involving unusually levels of oxidative stress. The object here is to point out the need and value of biomarkers of oxidative stress both for research and in the clinic. We have not included references, but these can be readily obtained on Medline or the NLM Gateway web site.

Aging Processes
    Normal aging
    Accelerated aging processes (segmental progeria-related diseases) as in
        Down's syndrome
    Genetically inherited diseases (hemochromatosis, thalassemia)
Heart and Cardiovascular Disease and
    Ischemia reperfusion injuries
    Atherosclerosis
    Adriamycin cardiotoxicity
    Alcohol cardiomyopathy
    Atherosclerotic cardiovascular events
Cancer Disease of All Tissues
Nervous System Dysfunctions
    Stroke and ischemia reperfusion injury
    Alzheimer's disease
    Parkinson's disease
    Neuronal ceroid lipofuscinoses
    Amyotrophic lateral Sclerosis (Lou Gehrig' s disease)
Muscle Dysfunctions
    Muscular dystrophy
    Multiple sclerosis
Eye
    Eye age-related macular degeneration
    Degenerative retinal damage
    Cataracts
Kidney
    Autoimmune nephrotic syndromes
    Heavy metal nephrotoxicity
    Chronic kidney disease
    Uremia

Gastrointestinal System
  Diabetes (type 1 and 2)
  Pancreatitis
  Hydrocarbon liver injury
  Inflammatory bowel disease
Lung
  Lung cancer (smoking)
  Emphysema
  Bronchopulmonary dysphasia
  Asbestos carcinogenicity
  Chronic obstructive pulmonary disease (COPD)
  Asthma
Hemopoietic System
  Sickle cell anemia
  Malaria
  Fanconi's anemia
  Human immunodeficiency virus disease
Liver
  Alcohol-induced liver cirrhosis
  Hepatitis B
Skin
  Porphyria
  Ultra violet skin damage
  Lichen sclerosus
Pregnancy
  Pre-eclampsia
Radiation mediated dysfunctions (ionization and non-ionization sources)
Age related disease associated with long term chronic inflammation

THE OXIDATIVE STRESS PROFILE CONCEPT

The hypothesis that needs to be more fully tested is that oxidative damage, as indicated by an individual's oxidative stress index, is indicative of a person's risk to disease and possibly accelerated aging processes. Thus, any lowering of this oxidative stress index would be expected to result in some degree of long-term benefit in promoting extended health and productive longevity for that individual. This argument is made stronger by the use of assays that have already shown health and longevity correlations. However, lowering an individual's oxidative stress status to a given degree may be more beneficial to some individuals than others. We are not aware of any evidence that suggests that lowering oxidative damage in an individual will have some harmful effect.

Thus, the more pertinent question may be: How much benefit will accrue with a given degree of lowered oxidative stress? Clearly, an answer to that question will come only after many more and long-term studies. However, a number of experts in the field are now becoming increasingly convinced that oxidative stress is important as a marker of general health status and that useful markers of oxidative stress are now available for use to further test these concepts. One could argue that if we can lower an individual's oxidative stress status without any harmful side effect at a reasonable cost, then why not do it?[92–97]

Here, we think the greatest potential problems are the natural biovariations that occur within an individual over time. These problems can be reduced to some degree by controlling the time and diet variables, but it is clearly of key importance to select those assays having minimal biovariations.[92,94–96,98–102]

DEVELOPMENT OF THE OXIDATIVE STRESS PROFILE

Since many papers have been published over the past year on the use of biomarkers of oxidative stress, it appears reasonable to select the assays best supported in the scientific literature.[55,91,103,104] We believe there are advantages to choosing those assays that have successfully shown a correlation with age and longevity (preferably in human or other primate species).

Another advantage would be to select those assays that can use samples collected non-invasively: blood (serum, plasma, RBC pellet, and lymphocyte), urine (24-hr, overnight fast, first morning void) and breath (taken before and after a controlled exercise about 70% VO_{max}.).

Although there is a need for simplicity and lower costs there is no one single assay yet known that can assess oxidative status of an individual using any of the listed non-invasive samples available. There is also the problem of assays having unique interfering reactions in samples and different degrees of accuracy, precision, and biovariation. Thus, multi-assays measuring a given class of oxidative stress is recommended until better assays become available.[105–108] Clearly cost, difficulty of assay, precision, accuracy, biovariation, and throughput efficiency are other key factors to evaluate in choosing an array of markers of oxidative stress.[2,55,91,104,109]

It should also be pointed out that the data obtained from all overnight urine collection assays usually always need to be normalized to correct for differences in water consumption and lean body mass of the different individuals being measured. Such normalization is not necessary for a 24-hour collection protocol, but such a sample is more difficult to obtain and recent studies have found no statistical differences.

A standard protocol requires the freezing and thawing of urine and serum samples. When measuring 8-OHdG in urine, it is essential to heat the urine sample (typically 20 minutes at 40°C) to free the DNA damage product from phosphate precipitant. All fat-soluble analytes measured in a serum sample should be normalized by the fat content of the serum.[110–113] For example, for the tocopherols, total lipid is calculated from the triglyceride and cholesterol values of the blood sample. Whether such normalization is also needed for vitamin A and the other carotenoids is still controversial. Isoprostane data should be normalized against BMI to correct for total fat difference. This recommendation is based on the positive correlation reported between isoprostane values and BMI in subjects.

Long-term high-level reproducibility is essential since patients will return on a monthly, quarterly, or yearly basis, and thus internal standards must be in place to assure accurate comparative results for the patient on each return visit. This requires stable internal control samples, where correction of data is allowed with reference to these internal and external standards. To achieve these results, the quality of the laboratory running these assays needs to be higher than usual for a regular reference laboratory that does not have the same goals for their tests.

PROPOSED ASSAYS FOR THE OXIDATIVE STRESS PROFILE

The following consist of a list of biomarkers of oxidative stress and includes both markers of damage and antioxidants. They were taken from a recent survey of the literature and reasonably represent what the current scientific communities in this field are using successfully.

A. Oxidative Damage (blood, urine, and breath)

(a) Nucleic acids (urine)
  8-hydroxy-2-deoyguanosine (8OHdG)
  5-hydroxy-methyluracil (5OHmU)
  8-oxo-guanosine (8oxoGuo)

(b) Lipids (urine)
  8-epe-PGF2-alpha isoprostane
  2,3-dinor 8-PGF2-alpha (2,3-dinor isoprostane
  Alkenyls (malonaldehyde and 4-hydroynonenal)
  Hydroperoxides I (aqueous)

(c) Lipids (serum)
  Alkenyls (malonaldehyde and 4-hydroynonenal)
  Hydroperoxides II (lipid)
  Oxidized LDL

(d) Proteins (serum)
Protein carbonyls (dityrosine and nitrotyrosine)

B. Protective/Defense Processes (Antioxidants)

(a) Endogenous (serum)
Albumin
Bilirubin
Ceruloplasmin
Total thiols
Uric acid
Metallothionein
Thioredoxin
Lipoic acid
Lipid peroxidation inhibition capacity (LPIC)

(b) Exogenous (serum)
Ascorbate
Carotenoids (8)
Tocopherols (3)
Coenzyme Q10

(c) Oxygen Radical Absorption Capacity (ORAC) (serum)
Total
Aqueous
Lipid

(d) Iron Profile (serum)
Total iron
Available iron-binding capacity(AIBC)
Total binding capacity(TIBC)
Percent iron saturation (total iron/TIBC) X 100
Ferritin

(e) Glycation Status (serum)
Glucose
Glycated protein (fructosamine)

(f) Trace metal analysis
(22 elements analyzed by inductive coupled plasma-mass spectrometry
(ICP) and separated into antioxidant, pro-oxidant and toxic classes.

(C) Markers of Inflammation (serum)

C-reactive protein (CPR)
Heat-shock protein (HSP70)
Myeloperoxidase (MPO)
Tumor necrosis factor alpha (TNF-alpha)
Interleukin-1

Interleukin-6
Interleukin-18
Heme oxidase-1 (HO-1)
Bcl-2

VALIDATION OF THE OXIDATIVE STRESS

From our limited studies we have found a large range of oxidative stress status in different individuals. However, very few of these individuals were actually significantly far from the mean. In turn we found that those individuals that had unusually high oxidative stress status were usually the major responders to antioxidant dietary supplementation. Most all other individuals showed very little if any response to dietary supplementation of antioxidants. It is also important to note that we could never get a person's OSS to super-low levels; the best that sould be achieved is to bring the levels close to normalcy.

Thus, it appears that oxidative stress is controlled and regulated in humans and probably other organisms around a given set point, and that this set point is maintained over a larger range of diets, lifestyles, exercise, and environmental exposures. It appears that when these oxidative stress regulators are not functioning properly then antioxidant supplementation works.

In a clinical study where individuals are given an antioxidant supplement without a previous screening test, it is thus not surprising to learn that the response to increased protection to a given disease is largely negative. This is because most of the time the person's oxidative stress status was not affected by the antioxidant supplement. A similar conclusion was recently reported by Balz Frei.[92,114-116]

DEVELOPMENT OF AN OXIDATIVE STRESS PROFILE REPORT

Because an oxidative stress profile report is more complex than a typical reference laboratory report, more effort is required in its design if the data are to be understood by the physician as well as by the patient. Thus the report needs to be functional, but at the same time easy to understand. We recommend showing the results both in absolute values and on a percentile basis. The use of percentiles allows the integration (percent of average values for that assay) of different assays having different units of measurement. This would be valuable if an objective was to arrive at a general oxidative stress index or antioxidant index reflecting the summation of all the different tests used. There are some advantages in the medical community to keep the final results simple, and if the oxidative stress profile consists of some 20 or more parameters, the index strategy may prove to be useful.

The validity of the assays used could be evaluated by calculation of an oxidative stress index (OSI) and an antioxidant index (AOI) and then plotting them against each other. An inverse relation would be expected, which could then, in theory, be refined by calculating weight factors for each test result to optimize the negative correlation.

The oxidative stress profile procedure would also greatly benefit if data from other tests unrelated to oxidative stress were included. This procedure would allow a more complete assessment of a patient's functional status and would further assist the physician in identifying possible recommended treatments and therapies. The following list suggests what additional profiles we have found useful in this regard:

Hormone profile
Trace metal profile
Cardiovascular risk factor profile
Liver function profile
Kidney function profile
Glucose resistance/insulin/IGF-1 profile

General physical health examination should include an O_2V_{max} value and results of cognitive function and memory tests.

USE OF THE OXIDATIVE STRESS PROFILE IN AN OPTIMAL HEALTH PROGRAM

Assuming that the patient is generally in good health, the object of the oxidative stress profile is to provide the physician with sufficient information to minimize the patient's long-term oxidative stress status. This is achieved by utilizing the principle of "feedback loop" between patient and physician. That is, there need to be frequent follow-up tests to determine how the recommended therapy is working.

This is exactly the same process as when the physician wants the patient to reach a certain cholesterol level. This procedure has the very important benefit that the patient gains information on the basis of recommended treatment by the physician, and then first-hand knowledge of the data on a return visit if the treatment is actually working. Since even successful lowering of an individual's oxidative stress status is not perceived (they rarely feel any better), then the use of the oxidative stress profiles in a clinical setting needs such a feedback loop for "customer satisfaction."

In theory. then, the oxidative stress profile procedure could provide an individual with information of whether he needs to take any antioxidant supplement or decrease eating certain foods (for example, those that are high in iron). If such supplements are indicated, then the patient would know why such dietary supplements are advocated and in the amounts recommended. The big payoff is, however, when the regimen works for the patient. That is, if on a return visit oxidative stress is lowered and on several other return visits a diet is reached such that the patient has "peaked out." This is like finding out that the therapy actually did lower a patient's cholesterol. It is this personalized approach to the control of a patient's oxidative stress status that is a key component of the oxidative stress profile approach. Right now, millions of individuals are taking antioxidant supplements, without knowing whether they are taking the right ones and in the right amount, and, of course, whether they are working at all.

SUMMARY AND CONCLUSION

Information is steadily growing in the field of free radicals in biology and medicine, indicating the general importance of oxidative stress and related inflammation disorders to human health and longevity. There is also an increasing need to translate this knowledge to practical applications for the human population. In this paper, we briefly review some of the progress in this field and propose the development of an oxidative stress profile as an approach in personalized medicine to help accelerate the practical application of this knowledge.

Many problems need to be solved in the development of the oxidative stress profile, but our own experience to date with this approach has indicated that the basic concept appears sound.

ACKNOWLEDGMENTS

We would like to thank the members of Exeter Life Sciences, the Green Light Committee and the Kronos Longevity Research Institute for their continued encouragement and support.

REFERENCES

1. HALLIWELL, B. 1996. Antioxidants in human health and disease. Annu. Rev. Nutr. **16:** 33–50.
2. CUTLER, R.G. & H. RODRIGUEZ. 2003. Critical Reviews of Oxidative Stress and Aging: Advances in Basic Science, Diagnostics and Intervention. World Scientific. Singapore.
3. CUTLER, R.G. 1995. Oxidative Stress and Aging. Molecular and Cell Biology Updates. Birkhauser Verlag. Boston and Basel.

4. WEI, Y.H. & H.C. LEE. 2002. Oxidative stress, mitochondrial DNA mutation, and impairment of antioxidant enzymes in aging. Exp. Biol. Med. (Maywood) **227:** 671–682.

5. BARJA, G. 2002. Rate of generation of oxidative stress-related damage and animal longevity. Free Radic. Biol. Med. **33:** 1167–1172.

6. LENAZ, G. *et al.* 1999. Mitochondria, oxidative stress, and antioxidant defences. Acta Biochim. Pol. **46:** 1–21.

7. BARJA, G. 1999. Mitochondrial oxygen radical generation and leak: sites of production in states 4 and 3, organ specificity, and relation to aging and longevity. J. Bioenerg. Biomembr. **31:** 347–366.

8. AUSTAD, S.N. 1997. Comparative aging and life histories in mammals. Exp. Gerontol. **32:** 23–38.

9. CUTLER, R.G. 1996. The molecular and evolutionary aspects of human aging and longevity. *In* Advances in Anti-Aging Medicine. R. Klatz, Ed.: 71–99. Mary Ann Liebert. New York.

10. KIRKWOOD, T.L., P. KAPAHI & D.P. SHANLEY. 2000. Evolution, stress, and longevity. J. Anat. **197:** 587–590.

11. NESSE, R.M. & G.C. WILLIAMS. 1998. Evolution and the origins of disease. Sci. Am. **279:** 86–93.

12. GAVRILOV, L.A. & N.S. GAVRILOVA. 2002. Evolutionary theories of aging and longevity. ScientificWorldJournal **2:** 339–356.

13. HAMILTON, W.D. 1966. The moulding of senescence by natural selection. J. Theor. Biol. **12:** 12–45.

14. AUSTAD, S.N. 1997. Why We Age: What Science is Discovering about the body's journey through life. J. Wiley & Sons. New York.

15. KIRKWOOD, T.B.L. 1999. Time of Our Lives: The Science of Human Aging. Oxford University Press. New York.

16. CUTLER, R.G. 1976. Nature of aging and life maintenance processes. *In* Interdisciplinary Topics in Gerontology. R.G. Cutler, Ed.: 83–133. S. Karger: Basel.

17. CUTLER, R.G. 1978. Evolutionary biology of senescence. *In* The Biology of Aging, J.A. Behnke, C.E. Finch & G.B. Moment, Eds: 311–360. Plenum: New York.

18. ROSE, M.R. & C.E. FINCH. 1994. Genetics and Evolution of Aging. Contemporary Issues in Genetics and Evolution, Vol 3: 311–360. Kluwer. Dordrecht and Boston.

19. SOHAL, R.S., B.H. SOHAL & W.C. ORR. 1995. Mitochondrial superoxide and hydrogen peroxide generation, protein oxidative damage, and longevity in different species of flies. Free Radic. Biol. Med. **19:** 499–504.

20. LIBBY, P. & P.M. RIDKER. 2004. Inflammation and atherosclerosis: role of C-reactive protein in risk assessment. Am. J. Med. **116:** 9S–16S.

21. FINCH, C.E. & E.M. CRIMMINS. 2004. Inflammatory exposure and historical changes in human life-spans. Science **305:** 1736–1739.

22. GIRMAN, C.J. *et al.* 2004. The metabolic syndrome and risk of major coronary events in the Scandinavian Simvastatin Survival Study (4S) and the Air Force/Texas Coronary Atherosclerosis Prevention Study (AFCAPS/TexCAPS). Am. J. Cardiol. **93:** 136–141.

23. ERLINGER, T.P. *et al.* 2004. C-reactive protein and the risk of incident colorectal cancer. JAMA **291:** 585–590.

24. BECKMAN, K.B. & B.N. AMES. 1998. The free radical theory of aging matures. PhysiolRev **78:** 547–581.
25. HARMAN, D. 1956. Aging: a theory based on free radical and radiation chemistry. J. Gerontol. **11:** 298–300.
26. HARMAN, D. & L.H. PIETTE. 1966. Free radical theory of aging: free radical reactions in serum. J. Gerontol. 1966. **21:** 560–565.
27. HARMAN, D. 1969. Prolongation of life: role of free radical reactions in aging. J. Am. Geriatr. Soc. **17:** 721–735.
28. HARMAN, D. 1998. Aging: phenomena and theories. Ann. N.Y. Acad. Sci. **854:** 1–7.
29. FINKEL, T. & N.J. HOLBROOK. 2000. Oxidants, oxidative stress and the biology of ageing. Nature **408:** 239–247.
30. GUARENTE, L. & C. KENYON. 2000. Genetic pathways that regulate ageing in model organisms. Nature **408:** 255–262.
31. GRAY, D.A. 2003. Strategies for engineered negligible senescence. Sci. Aging Knowledge Environ. **2003:** 30.
32. CUTLER, R.G. 1972. Transcription of reiterated DNA sequence classes throughout the life-span of the mouse. *In* Advances in Gerontological Research. B.S. Strehler, Ed.: 220–340. Academic Press. New York.
33. CUTLER, R.G. 1982. The dysdifferentiative hypothesis of mammalian aging and longevity. *In* The Aging Brain Cellular and Molecular Mechanisms of Aging in the Nervous System. G.F. E. Giacobini & A. Vernadakis, Eds.: 1–19. Raven Press. New York.
34. CUTLER, R.G. 1982. Longevity is determined by specific genes: testing the hypothesis. *In* Testing the Theories of Aging. R. Adelman & G. Roth, Eds.: 25–114. CRC Press. Boca Raton, FL.
35. CUTLER, R.G. 1991. Recent progress in testing the longevity determinant and dysdifferentiation hypotheses of aging. Arch. Gerontol. Geriatr. **12:** 75–98.
36. CUTLER, R.G. 1992. Genetic stability and oxidative stress: common mechanisms in aging and cancer. Exs **62:** 31–46.
37. DEAN, R.G., S.H. SOCHER & R.G. CUTLER. 1985. Dysdifferentiative nature of aging: age-dependent expression of mouse mammary tumor virus and casein genes in brain and liver tissues of the C57BL/6J mouse strain. Arch. Gerontol. Geriatr. **4:** 43–51.
38. CUTLER, R. 1992. Genetic stability and oxidative stress: common mechanisms in aging and cancer. *In* Free Radicals and Aging. I. Emerit & B. Chance, Eds.: 31–46. Birkhauer Verlag. Basel
39. CUTLER, R.G. 1991. Recent progress in testing the longevity determinant and dysdifferentiation hypothesis of aging. Arch. Gerontol. Geriat. **12:** 75–98.
40. ARMSTRONG, R.J. & C.N. SVENDSEN. 2000. Neural stem cells: from cell biology to cell replacement. Cell Transplant. **9:** 139–152.
41. EDELSTEIN-KESHET, L., A. ISRAEL & P. LANSDORP. 2001. Modelling perspectives on aging: can mathematics help us stay young? J. Theor. Biol. **213:** 509–525.
42. GALVIN, K.A. & D.G. JONES. 2002. Adult human neural stem cells for cell-replacement therapies in the central nervous system. Med. J. Aust. **177:** 316–318.
43. ZARET, K. 2004. Regenerative medicine: self-help for insulin cells. Nature **429:** 30–31.
44. REYA, T. *et al.* 2001. Stem cells, cancer, and cancer stem cells. Nature **414:** 105–111.

45. EGGER, G. *et al.* 2004. Epigenetics in human disease and prospects for epigenetic therapy. Nature **429:** 457–463.
46. JONES, P.A. 2003. Epigenetics in carcinogenesis and cancer prevention. Ann. N.Y. Acad. Sci. **983:** 213–219.
47. JONES, P.A. & P.W. LAIRD. 1999. Cancer epigenetics comes of age. Nat. Genet. **21:** 163–167.
48. JONES, P.A. & D. TAKAI. 2001. The role of DNA methylation in mammalian epigenetics. Science **293:** 1068–1070.
49. CUTLER, R.G. 1975. Evolution of human longevity and the genetic complexity governing aging rate. Proc. Natl. Acad. Sci. USA **72:** 4664–4668.
50. ASIF, M. *et al.* 2000. An advanced glycation endproduct cross-link breaker can reverse age-related increases in myocardial stiffness. Proc. Natl. Acad. Sci. USA **97:** 2809–2813.
51. OTURAI, P.S. *et al.* 2000. Effects of advanced glycation end-product inhibition and cross-link breakage in diabetic rats. Metabolism **49:** 996–1000.
52. RAJ, D.S. *et al.* 2000. Advanced glycation end products: a nephrologist's perspective. Am. J. Kidney Dis. **35:** 365–380.
53. STITT, A. *et al.* 2002. The AGE inhibitor pyridoxamine inhibits development of retinopathy in experimental diabetes. Diabetes **51:** 2826–2832.
54. VLASSARA, H., M. BROWNLEE & A. CERAMI. 1986. Nonenzymatic glycosylation: role in the pathogenesis of diabetic complications. Clin. Chem. **32:** B37–41.
55. HALLIWELL, B. & J.M.C. GUTTERIDGE. 1999. Free radicals in biology and medicine, 3rd ed. Oxford University Press. New York.
56. WILLIAMS, G.M., Ed. 1993. Advances in Modern Environmental Toxicology. Princeton Scientific Publishing. Princeton, NJ.
57. AUST, O. *et al.* 2003. Lycopene oxidation product enhances gap junctional communication. Food Chem. Toxicol. **41:** 1399–1407.
58. CRANE, F.L. 2001. Biochemical functions of coenzyme Q10. J. Am. Coll. Nutr. **20:** 591–598.
59. CUTLER, R.G. 1984. Urate and ascorbate: their possible roles as antioxidants in determining longevity of mammalian species. Arch. Gerontol. Geriatr. **3:** 321–348.
60. CUTLER, R.G. 1985. Antioxidants and longevity of mammalian species. *In* Molecular Biology of Aging. A.D.B.A.D. Woodhead & A. Hollaender, Eds. :15–74. Plenum Press. New York.
61. CUTLER, R.G. 1991. Antioxidants and aging. Am. J. Clin. Nutr. **53**(1 Suppl): 373S–379S.
62. GAREWAL, H.S. 1997. Antioxidants and Disease Prevention. CRC Press. Boca Raton, FL.
63. HADLEY, C.W. *et al.* 2002. Tomatoes, lycopene, and prostate cancer: progress and promise. Exp. Biol. Med. (Maywood) **227:** 869–880.
64. LITTARRU, G.P. & R. BELARDINELLI. 2004. Effect of CoQ-10 administration on myocardial function and vascular response in ischemic heart disease. Toxicol. Ind. Hlth. Vol. 9.
65. MARTIN-GALLAN, P. *et al.* 2003. Biomarkers of diabetes-associated oxidative stress and antioxidant status in young diabetic patients with or without subclinical complications. Free Radic. Biol. Med. **34:** 1563–1574.
66. MEYDANI, M. 1992. Vitamin E requirement in relation to dietary fish oil and oxidative stress in elderly. Exs **62:** 411–418.

67. NIETO, F.J. *et al.* 2000. Uric acid and serum antioxidant capacity: a reaction to atherosclerosis? Atherosclerosis **148**: 131–139.
68. OSGANIAN, S.K. *et al.* 2003. Dietary carotenoids and risk of coronary artery disease in women. Am. J. Clin. Nutr. **77**: 1390–1399.
69. CESARATTO, L. *et al.* 2004. The importance of redox state in liver damage. Ann. Hepatol. **3**: 86–92.
70. JOHNSON, E.J. 2005. Obesity, lutein metabolism, and age-related macular degeneration: a web of connections. Nutr. Rev. **63**: 9–15.
71. TIRANATHANAGUL, K. *et al.* 2004. Oxidative stress from rapid versus slow intravenous iron replacement in haemodialysis patients. Nephrology (Carlton) **9**: 217–222.
72. MERRY, B.J. 2004. Oxidative stress and mitochondrial function with aging: the effects of calorie restriction. Aging Cell **3**: 7–12.
73. CAIMI, G., C. CAROLLO & R. LO PRESTI. 2003. Diabetes mellitus: oxidative stress and wine. Curr. Med. Res. Opin. **19**: 581–586.
74. TOESCU, V. *et al.* 2002. Oxidative stress and normal pregnancy. Clin. Endocrinol. (Oxf) **57**: 609–613.
75. POLIDORI, M.C. *et al.* 2001.Profiles of antioxidants in human plasma. Free Radic. Biol. Med. **30**: 456–462.
76. SODHI, C.P. *et al.* 1997. Study of oxidative-stress in rifampicin-induced hepatic injury in growing rats with and without protein-energy malnutrition. Hum. Exp. Toxicol. **16**: 315–321.
77. CADENAS, E. & H. SIES. 1985. Oxidative stress: excited oxygen species and enzyme activity. Adv. Enzyme Regul. **23**: 217–237.
78. SIES, H. & E. CADENAS. 1985. Oxidative stress: damage to intact cells and organs. Phil. Trans. R. Soc. Lond., B Biol. Sci. **311**: 617–631.
79. SIES, H. 1991. Oxidative stress: from basic research to clinical application. Am. J. Med. **91**: 31S–38S.
80. SIES, H. 1991. Role of reactive oxygen species in biological processes. Klin. Wochenschr. **69**: p. 965–968.
81. SIES, H. 1997. Oxidative stress: oxidants and antioxidants. Exp. Physiol. **82**: 291–295.
82. SIES, H. 1985. Oxidative Stress. Academic Press. Orlando, FL.
83. TOLMASOFF, J.M., T. ONO & R.G. CUTLER. 1980. Superoxide dismutase: correlation with life-span and specific metabolic rate in primate species. Proc. Natl. Acad. Sci. USA **77**: 2777–2781.
84. MADEBO, T. *et al.* 2003. Circulating antioxidants and lipid peroxidation products in untreated tuberculosis patients in Ethiopia. Am. J. Clin. Nutr. **78**: 117–122.
85. MARCOVINA, S.M., V.P. GAUR & J.J. ALBERS. 1994. Biological variability of cholesterol, triglyceride, low- and high-density lipoprotein cholesterol, lipoprotein(a), and apolipoproteins A-I and B. Clin. Chem. **40**: 574–578.
86. HELMERSSON, J. & S. BASU. 1999. F2-isoprostane excretion rate and diurnal variation in human urine. Prostaglandins Leukot. Essent. Fatty Acids. **61**: 203–205.
87. YU, X., C.S. HO & C.W. LAM. 2004. Biological variation of plasma F2-isoprostane-III and arachidonic acid in healthy individuals. Clin. Chem. **50**: 1428–1430.
88. COVAS, M.I. *et al.* 1997. Biological variation of superoxide dismutase in erythrocytes and glutathione peroxidase in whole blood. Clin. Chem. **43**: 1991–1993.

89. SCHECTMAN, G., M. PATSCHES & E.A. SASSE. 1996. Variability in cholesterol measurements: comparison of calculated and direct LDL cholesterol determinations. Clin. Chem. **42:** 732–737.

90. KAFONEK, S.D. *et al.* 1996. Biological variation of lipids and lipoproteins in fingerstick blood. Clin. Chem. **42:** 2002–2007.

91. PACKER, L. & J. YODOI. 1993. Redox regulation of cell signaling and its clinical application. *In* Oxidative stress and disease. Marcel Dekker. New York

92. FREI, B. 2004. Efficacy of dietary antioxidants to prevent oxidative damage and inhibit chronic disease. J. Nutr. **134:** 3196S–3198S.

93. CARR, A.C. & B. FREI. 1999. Toward a new recommended dietary allowance for vitamin C based on antioxidant and health effects in humans. Am. J. Clin. Nutr. **69:** 1086–1107.

94. CHEN, K. *et al.* 2000. Vitamin C suppresses oxidative lipid damage in vivo, even in the presence of iron overload. Am. J. Physiol. Endocrinol. Metab. **279:** E1406–1412.

95. FREI, B. 1999. On the role of vitamin C and other antioxidants in atherogenesis and vascular dysfunction. Proc. Soc. Exp. Biol. Med. **222:** 196–204.

96. MCCALL, M.R. & B. FREI. 1999. Can antioxidant vitamins materially reduce oxidative damage in humans? Free Radic. Biol. Med. **26:** 1034–1053.

97. SUH, J.H. *et al.* 2001. Oxidative stress in the aging rat heart is reversed by dietary supplementation with (R)-(alpha)-lipoic acid. FASEB J. **15:** 700-706.

98. BERGER, T.M. *et al.* 1997. Antioxidant activity of vitamin C in iron-overloaded human plasma. J. Biol. Chem. **272:** 15656–15660.

99. DUFFY, S.J. *et al.* 2001. Short- and long-term black tea consumption reverses endothelial dysfunction in patients with coronary artery disease. Circulation **104:** 151–156.

100. GOKCE, N. *et al.* 1999. Long-term ascorbic acid administration reverses endothelial vasomotor dysfunction in patients with coronary artery disease. Circulation **99:** 3234–3240.

101. BLUMBERG, J. 2004. Use of biomarkers of oxidative stress in research studies. J. Nutr. **134:** 3188S–3189S.

102. SEIFRIED, H.E. *et al.* 2004. Free radicals: the pros and cons of antioxidants: executive summary report. J. Nutr. **134:** 3143S–3163S.

103. PACKER, L., M. HIRAMATSU & T. YOSHIKAWA. 1999. Antioxidant food supplements in human health.: Academic Press. San Dieg, CA.

104. ARMSTRONG, D. 1998. Free radical and antioxidant protocols. Humana Press. Totowa, NJ.

105. NIA, A.B. *et al.* 2001. A multi-biomarker approach to study the effects of smoking on oxidative DNA damage and repair and antioxidative defense mechanisms. Carcinogenesis **22:** 395–401.

106. JACKSON, M.J. 1999. An overview of methods for assessment of free radical activity in biology. Proc. Nutr. Soc. **58:** 1001–1006.

107. KHASSAF, M. *et al.* 2003. Effect of vitamin C supplements on antioxidant defence and stress proteins in human lymphocytes and skeletal muscle. J. Physiol. **549:** 645–652.

108. ORHAN, H. *et al.* 2004. Evaluation of a multi-parameter biomarker set for oxidative damage in man: increased urinary excretion of lipid, protein and DNA oxidation products after one hour of exercise. Free Radic. Biol. Med. **38:** 1269–1279.

109. GREENWALD, R.A. 1985. CRC Handbook of Methods for Oxygen Radical Research. CRC Press. Boca Raton, FL.
110. MERAJI, S. *et al.* 2000. Relationship between classic risk factors, plasma antioxidants and indicators of oxidant stress in angina pectoris (AP) in Tehran. Atherosclerosis **150:** 403–412.
111. JORDAN, P. *et al.* 1997. Modelling of mortality data from a multi-centre study in Japan by means of Poisson regression with error in variables. Int. J. Epidemiol. **26:** 501–507.
112. GEY, K.F. 1995. Cardiovascular disease and vitamins: Concurrent correction of "suboptimal" plasma antioxidant levels may, as important part of "optimal" nutrition, help to prevent early stages of cardiovascular disease and cancer, respectively. Bibl. Nutr. Dieta **1995(52):** 75–91.
113. GEY, K.F. 1994. Optimum plasma levels of antioxidant micronutrients: ten years of antioxidant hypothesis on arteriosclerosis. Bibl. Nutr. Dieta **1994(51):** 84-99.
114. FREI, B. & J.V. HIGDON, 2003. Antioxidant activity of tea polyphenols in vivo: evidence from animal studies. J. Nutr. **133:** 3275S–3284S.
115. WIDLANSKY, M.E. *et al.* 2005. Effects of black tea consumption on plasma catechins and markers of oxidative stress and inflammation in patients with coronary artery disease. Free Radic. Biol. Med. **38:** 499–506.
116. MASTALOUDIS, A. *et al.* 2004. Endurance exercise results in DNA damage as detected by the comet assay. Free Radic. Biol. Med. **36:** 966–975.

Controversies in Dyslipidemias

Atheroprevention in Diabetes and Insulin Resistance

ELIOT A. BRINTON

Metabolism Section, Cardiovascular Genetics, University of Utah School of Medicine, Salt Lake City, Utah, USA

ABSTRACT: Cardiovascular disease (CVD) is the leading cause of morbidity and mortality in industrialized countries. Patients with diabetes and insulin resistance are at even greater risk than the general population. Risk factors may be even more significant in predicting risk of disease when present in diabetic patients. Interaction among the elements of the metabolic syndrome/insulin resistance (MS/IR) in atherogenesis is currently the subject of much research. Efforts to understand the elements of the dyslipidemias associated with MS/IR are now beginning to pay off. An increasing number of drugs and other interventions have been shown to be effective in clinical trials in reducing risk factors and improving outcomes. The advantages and disadvantages of possible treatments of these dyslipidemias, including the risks and benefits of combination therapy, are discussed in detail. Finally, strategies for maintaining glucose control and the role of inflammation associated with MS/IR and CVD are described.

KEYWORDS: atherogenesis; diabetes; glucose tolerance; insulin resistance; cardiovascular disease; lipids; lipoproteins; trigylcerides; statins; cardiac risk factors; inflammation; metabolic syndrome; estrogen; obesity

ATHEROGENESIS IN DIABETES AND INSULIN RESISTANCE

There are about 16 million individuals with diabetes in the United States, a majority of whom have been diagnosed already. However, although it is about three times more common, insulin resistance is almost never diag-

Address for correspondence: Eliot A. Brinton, M.D., Cardiology Division, University of Utah, Room 4A100, 30 North 1900 East, Salt Lake City, Utah 84132. Voice: 801-581-3888; fax: 801-581-7715.

eliot@ucbg.med.utah.edu

Ann. N.Y. Acad. Sci. 1055: 159–178 (2005). © 2005 New York Academy of Sciences.
doi: 10.1196/annals.1323.024

Cholesterol Predicts CHD Mortality Rate in Diabetic and Nondiabetic Men
Multiple Risk Factor Intervention Trial (MRFIT)

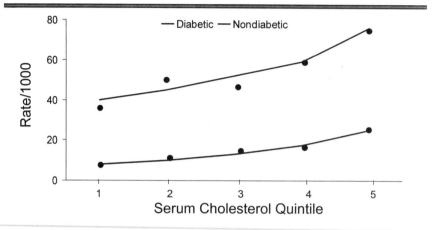

FIGURE 1. Coronary heart disease (CHD) event rates by quintile in persons with and without diabetes. Data from the Multiple Risk Factor Intervention Trial (MRFIT). (From Bierman, E.L. 1992. George Lyman Duff Memorial Lecture: atherogenesis in diabetes. Arterioscler. Thromb. **12:** 647–656. Reprinted with permission.)

nosed. The increase in risk of cardiovascular disease (CVD) is high in both cases, and the many mechanisms of this increase are similar.

The fact that diabetes increases the risk of atherosclerosis was demonstrated long ago, early in modern research into atherosclerosis, by the MR FIT (Multiple Risk Factor Intervention Trial).[1] FIGURE 1, taken from that study, shows coronary heart disease (CHD) event rates by quintile in persons with and without diabetes. Among the diabetes patients, even at a very low serum cholesterol level, the risk of a coronary event is perhaps twice as high as it is for a non-diabetic person who has a relatively high cholesterol level. There are two implications: (1) diabetes patients are always at added risk for atherosclerosis, whatever their other risk factors, and (2) factors other than total serum cholesterol and low-density lipoprotein (LDL) levels must contribute to atherosclerosis risk in diabetes patients.

FIGURE 2 shows results from the Bedford Study.[2] Note that diabetes mellitus erases the gender gap that favors women over men in age-matched CHD risk. Exactly why this is so is an interesting question that remains unanswered. The same phenomenon occurs in impaired glucose tolerance, and

Diabetes and glucose intolerance vs. cardiovascular mortality

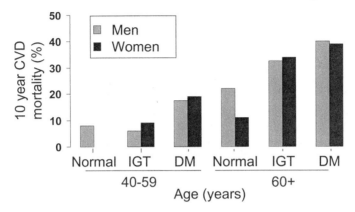

FIGURE 2. Diabetes and even impaired glucose intolerance (IGT) tend to eliminate the gender gap in which women have lower cardiovascular disease (CVD) risk than men at a given age. Also, the CVD risk in IGT is significantly elevated, midway between the risk with and without diabetes. Results from the Bedford Study[2] reprinted with permission.

Interrelationship Between Obesity, IR, DM and Atherosclerosis

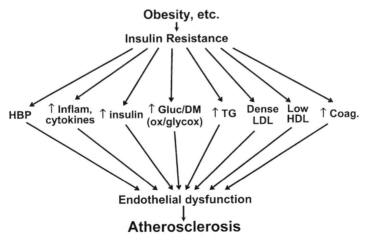

FIGURE 3. Simplified schema showing both hypothesized and established interrelationships among central adiposity, insulin resistance and atherosclerosis.

probably also in insulin resistance or the metabolic syndrome. In addition, the results show that the overall increase in CHD risk is almost as high for impaired glucose tolerance as it is for full-blown diabetes. The reason for this likely has to do with the factors shown in FIGURE 3. Removing hyperglycemia from the risk-factor equation leaves elevated blood pressure, accelerated inflammation, hyperinsulinemia, hypertriglyceridemia, low HDL levels, a hypercoagulable state, and, as discussed previously, small dense LDL particles. Absent diabetes, the remaining factors are still linked with atherosclerosis. This demonstrates the need for aggressive efforts to prevent atherosclerosis not only in diabetes, but also in the insulin-resistant patient who does not have diabetes.

There are many ways to determine whether someone has insulin resistance. The ATP-III guidelines (National Cholesterol Education Program, Third Report of the Expert Panel on Detection, Evaluation, and Treatment of High Blood Cholesterol in Adults)[3] referred to it as the metabolic syndrome, but I prefer the more specific term *insulin-resistance syndrome*. A diagnosis of metabolic syndrome is defined by three or more of the following five criteria, four of which are routinely determined for most patients. Each criterion by itself is a risk factor for atherosclerosis, and having determined them all will establish whether or not a patient is insulin-resistant.

- Waist circumference: girth greater than 40 inches for men, greater than 35 inches for a woman. Simple belt size may be one way to gain this information, although it may be an underestimate.

- Abdominal obesity: a categorical variable that does not require an exact measurement in inches or centimeters, but can be determined by the patient's appearance. It can be assessed, however, by measuring the circumference halfway between the bony prominences of the bottom of the ribs and the top of the ischial tuberosity or pelvis, assuring that the patient is not holding the abdomen in.

- A fasting triglyceride level higher than 150mg/dL and HDL-C (cholesterol) levels below 40 mg/dL for men or below 50 mg/dL for women.

- Blood pressure higher than 130 mmHg (systolic) or 85 mmHg (diastolic), or current use of anti-hypertensive medicine.

- Fasting glucose levels higher than 110 mg/dL. (Since the American Diabetes Association has dropped its lower limit for impaired fasting glucose from 110 to 100 mg/dL, I now prefer to use the lower threshold for metabolic syndrome.)

An additional method of diagnosing insulin resistance is the measurement of a fasting insulin level. This is not a part of the official criteria, because it is not well standardized, but an elevated or even above-average insulin level is very suggestive of the condition.

Cumulative Distribution of Plasma TG Levels: LDL Phenotypes A and B

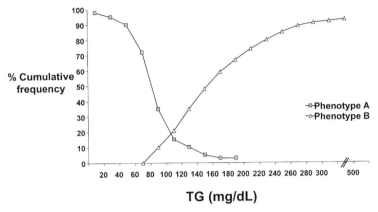

FIGURE 4. Cumulative distribution of plasma triglyceride levels: LDL phenotypes A and B. Third Report of the Expert Panel on Detection, Evaluation, and Treatment of High Blood Cholesterol in Adults (Adult Treatment Panel III) of the National Cholesterol Education Program.[3] Reprinted with permission.

LIPIDS AND ATHEROGENESIS IN DIABETES AND INSULIN RESISTANCE

Various lipid disorders appear to be related both to diabetes mellitus and to insulin resistance. First, a high triglyceride and low high-density lipoprotein (HDL) cholesterol level appear usually to coincide in all patients, and in individuals with diabetes and insulin resistance they are at least twice as prevalent as among other individuals. The current definition of metabolic syndrome by NCEP ATP III includes both of these parameters as two of the criteria.

FIGURE 4 shows the relationship between triglyceride (TG) level and small dense LDLs (phenotype B). Not only is there a strong positive relationship between TG levels and the prevalence of small dense LDLs, but this relationship increases very dramatically above a TG level in the mid- to lower 100s. According to the diagnostic criteria for metabolic syndrome, the lower cutoff for TGs is a level of 150 mg/dL, which is still relatively high, because between 100 and 150 mg/dL one begins to see a correlation with small dense LDLs and the other risk factors related to the metabolic syndrome.

There appear to be at least three direct mechanisms by which small dense LDLs may be atherogenic (see FIGURE 5):

- Smaller LDL particles can slip through the endothelial barrier more easily than other LDL particles. Circulating low-density lipoproteins probably cause little harm; only within the artery wall do they promote atherosclerosis.

- The atherogenicity of LDL is a function of the length of time it remains in the sub-endothelial matrix. The "dwell time," or stickiness, of an LDL particle is directly related to its size: Smaller particles remain longer in the sub-endothelial space.

- Even with equivalent dwell times, smaller LDL particles are more readily oxidized or otherwise modified, and modified LDL may be the ultimate driving force in atherogenesis.

By adhering to and migrating through the endothelium, modified LDL appears to drive the initial recruitment of inflammatory cells, their differentiation from monocyte to macrophage, and then the loading of cholesterol into the activated macrophage to form a macrophage foam cell. Thus small dense LDLs seem to drive central pathways in atherogenesis. In addition, small dense LDLs associate with other factors—insulin resistance, diabetes mellitus, low HDL, and high triglycerides—which of themselves are also probably

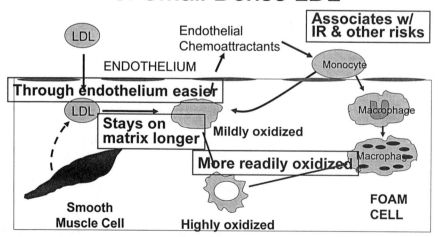

FIGURE 5. Extra atherogenicity of small dense LDL particles. *In vitro* studies suggest that small dense LDL particles enter into and adhere to the subendothelium more readily, and are more susceptible to oxidation, compared to large, buoyant LDLs.

atherogenic. With all these interconnections, it is no wonder that small dense LDLs are associated with increased CHD risk.

Another important problem related to small dense LDLs is a matter of recognition: Among patients with small dense LDLs, the customary LDL cholesterol level doubly underestimates their risk of CHD. Since each small dense LDL particle carries less cholesterol than other LDL particles, at an LDL of 100 a patient with small dense LDLs would have perhaps the equivalent of an LDL cholesterol of 110 or 120. This is still only marginally elevated above acceptable levels in the NCEP ATP III, but small, dense particles are also more atherogenic by nature. Thus a patient who has small dense LDLs and an LDL-C level of 99 mg/dL probably has a risk equivalent to that indicated by an LDL-C level of 130, 140, or possibly higher in another person who does not have small dense LDLs. Therefore the actual CHD risk may be very high in many insulin-resistant and diabetic patients who appear to have normal LDL cholesterol levels.

TESTING FOR SMALL DENSE LDLS

It is useful clinically to consider "extended" or "advanced" lipid profiles which measure more than just the standard lipid profile of total cholesterol, LDL-C, HDL-C and triglycerides. The benefit is largely to assess CHD risk correctly for a patient who may or may not have small dense LDLs. Also, looking at HDL particle size, as well as Lp(a) and remnant lipoprotein particle levels, may be helpful in making decisions about clinical management of atherosclerosis risk.

The criterion for ordering a special test is whether it will make a difference in treatment, and by that criterion in this patient population, the diagnosis of small dense LDLs is justified. I have already discussed the striking positive relationship between triglyceride levels and small dense LDLs, and there are equally striking data showing an inverse relationship between HDL cholesterol levels and small dense LDLs. A patient who has dramatically high triglyceride and/or low HDL levels has an overwhelming likelihood of having small dense LDLs, so one might not need to confirm its presence. However, about one-fourth of patients with small dense LDLs have triglyceride levels below 150 and an HDL-C level above 40 mg/dL, so it may be justified to measure LDL size directly in patients with normal TG and HDL levels, especially when the likelihood of small dense LDLs is intermediate.

Another setting in which an extended lipid profile could be useful is when further information is required about CHD risk. It is difficult to know how aggressively to treat a patient with intermediate risk who has not yet had a clinical event. In these cases, extra information can be very helpful to decide which treatment is appropriate. Another example is a patient who develops CHD but appears to have a normal lipid profile.

A third indication for measuring small dense LDLs is the presence of more severe coronary heart disease—more extensive atherosclerosis, or CHD at an earlier age—than the risk factors would predict. A related situation is progression of CHD despite what would appear to be adequate therapy.

Three types of extended or advanced lipid profiles are commercially available. The most widely available method, using gel electrophoresis, is provided by the Berkeley Heart Lab, but also can be set up to run in one's own lab, using the LipoPrint kit. Gel electrophoresis has been used for many years and is very well established. The Berkeley version of this method has been well-validated in a number of studies, but remains rather expensive despite some recent price reductions. Lipo-Science offers a new use of nuclear magnetic resonance (NMR) for clinical measurement of lipoprotein subfractions. The fact that this method measures lipoprotein subfractions by algorithmic deconvolution of complex signals, rather than by physical separation, worries many lipidologists, but it has been very well validated and correlated with atherosclerosis risk in a number of studies. It is more affordable than the Berkeley method, providing the complete panel with all the sub-fractions of LDL, VLDL, and HDL for a reasonable price. The LDL particle number is derived very indirectly from complicated algorithms. Although this number correlates strongly with CHD risk, it is not known whether it enhances CHD risk prediction by non-HDL-C or by total Apo B, which may be better measures of total atherogenic particles. Third, the vertical automated profile (VAP), offered by Atherotech, uses ultracentrifugation, a method developed at about the same time as gel electrophoresis, which also has been studied extensively and validated in a number of settings. VAP is CDC-standardized and is the most affordable of the three. In many clinical settings, a VAP costs the same as a basic lipid profile. Some practitioners obtain a VAP for every patient at every visit. Each of these tests is done in a single national center, so samples must be shipped out, but any laboratory that is able to send samples to reference laboratories can order these tests.

TREATMENT OPTIONS

There are numerous treatment possibilities for patients who have small dense LDL particles, but we are not certain of the relative value of these treatments. The best established, according to the clinical literature, is simply to lower LDL cholesterol further. Obviously, the statins are very useful for this purpose. Initiating statin treatment should be very effective in lowering LDL-C in a patient who has not been taking these medications. Generally, titrating the dose upward in a patient who is already taking a statin is less efficient, but it can still be helpful in lowering LDL-C further. Switching to a newer and more effective statin may also be useful, or one can consider combination therapy. Adding one of several other agents (niacin, the new cholesterol-absorption inhibitor ezetimibe, blue-acid sequestrants, and in some cases fenofibrate) may also be useful.

Instead of lowering LDL-C further, or more likely in addition, one can try to increase LDL particle size. Niacin may have the best effect of any available agent, but the fibrates are also useful in this regard. As a class, the statins are not very effective in increasing average LDL particle size, but some studies have suggested that some statins may have a modest favorable effect in this regard. The thiazoledinediones, a class of drugs used primarily for glycemic control and not for dyslipidemia, also are quite effective in increasing LDL particle size. It is still not certain that thiazoledinediones actually help prevent atherosclerotic events, but there is some evidence that these drugs may be effective for carotid intimal medial thickness. Clinical trials now under way may establish whether the thiazoledinediones are protective against atherogenesis.

Finally, one can treat insulin resistance, which is usually the root cause of the problem, starting with diet, exercise, weight loss, and medications. However, few practitioners are serious about prescribing diet and exercise, assuming that patients do not want to hear about them and will not comply. Furthermore, there is no reimbursement for instructing patients about these interventions, few doctors know how to teach patients about diet and exercise, and it is time-consuming to do so. Writing a prescription is far easier than talking to a patient about lifestyle. In addition, there is some controversy, especially with regard to diet, as to which approach is really the best. Nonetheless, it is imperative that we find an effective way to encourage patients to make the lifestyle changes needed to control insulin resistance.

As to pharmacological approaches, the thiazoledinediones (or TZDs) are well known to be excellent insulin-sensitizers. Metformin is a much weaker insulin-sensitizer, but it can be useful in particular settings such as polycystic ovary syndrome, which is a part of the complex of insulin resistance. Ramipril, an angiotensin-converting enzyme (ACE) inhibitor, was found in the HOPE (Heart Outcomes Prevention Evaluation) study[4] to reduce new cases of diabetes mellitus, though it is not clear that ACE inhibitors are truly insulin-sensitizers. A related class of drugs, angiotensin receptor blockers, also appears to have this effect. In neither case, however, is the mechanism of this effect well understood. The fibrates, which are PPAR-alpha agonists, are related to the thiazoledinediones, which are PPAR-gamma agonists, and they share some of the same actions, in that the TZDs have some lipid benefits similar to those of the fibrates. Thus the fibrates might help with insulin resistance. Several pharmaceutical companies are trying to develop agents that are both PPAR-alpha and -gamma agonists. It is not likely that the statins reduce insulin resistance or prevent diabetes; although one study suggested a reduction in incidence of new cases of diabetes with statin use, other studies have failed to confirm this.

GUIDELINES FOR LIPID REDUCTION IN DIABETES AND INSULIN RESISTANCE

TABLE 1 shows the current NCEP ATP-III guidelines. There are 3 LDL-C goals: levels of less than 160, 130, and 100 mg/dL, for low- and high-risk primary prevention, and secondary prevention, respectively. The latter is not just for coronary atherosclerosis, but includes atherosclerosis elsewhere in the body (primarily the carotid artery and lower extremities). These guidelines include diabetes as a CHD risk equivalent, as well as a Framingham global-risk score higher than 20% for 10 years. In any of those settings, the LDL cholesterol goal drops to less than 100 mg/dL.

When a patient has a Framingham score of 10–20% risk over 10 years, the intermediate risk category, it is often unclear whether to start aggressive pharamacotherapy or not. In such cases, it can be very helpful to obtain additional information, such as a calcium score, an advanced lipid profile, or a C-reactive protein level, to make a more informed treatment decision.

Although there is some evidence that the coronary calcium score by computed tomography (CT) might provide better risk assessment than the global risk score, the area under the ROC curve differed little, 0.71 versus 0.81 between the global risk score and the coronary calcium scores, respectively. The global risk score has been tested more extensively, and is quick, easy, and inexpensive. It is a sound basis for risk assessment, to which other tests can be added, as needed and desired.

The East–West study (FIG. 6) has received a great deal of attention. Although some studies have reached contrary conclusions, the concept is interesting. In most studies, the risk of future myocardial infarction (MI) in a person with Type 2 diabetes who has not had a prior MI is actually somewhat less than that in a non-diabetic, but in this particular study it was slightly higher.[5] In any case, the risk is close enough to consider diabetes to constitute a CHD risk equivalent, which justifies aggressive efforts to lower LDL-C levels below 100 mg/dL.

Obviously, a patient with diabetes and a prior MI has a much higher risk of future MI than does someone with diabetes and no prior disease, but the NCEP ATP-III guidelines fail to take this into account. Also, the American Diabetes Association guidelines, which have been revised since ATP-III was written, still fail to recommend any difference in LDL-C goal for primary vs. secondary prevention in diabetes. It is difficult to imagine why patients with and without CHD should be treated in exactly the same way. Another problem with both guidelines is their lack of guidance regarding LDL-C goals in insulin resistance or the metabolic syndrome.

In my opinion, the LDL-C goals within the NCEP ATP-III guidelines should be adjusted according to the patient's circumstances. First, very high-risk patients should be treated more aggressively than patients with average

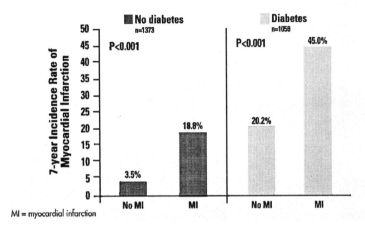

FIGURE 6. The risk of myocardial infarction in non-diabetics and diabetics, either with or without prior MI.[5] The *top bar* includes people with very little risk, intermediate risk, and higher risk, who have LDL cholesterol goals of 130 or 160 (by ATPIII guidelines). The *second bar* includes individuals at much higher risk whose LDL-C goal is lower, at 100. Reprinted with permission.

or borderline risk in a given category. Second, issues of quality of life and life expectancy should be taken into account. A patient who has everything to live for, is otherwise in excellent health, and for whom atherosclerosis is the rate-limiting step, deserves aggressive treatment. On the other hand, aggressive treatment is not justified in patients who are dying or are disabled from a different incurable disease. A third factor is whether the patient fears the treatment of atherosclerosis more than the atherosclerosis itself.

TABLE 1 comes from NCEP ATP-III. In primary prevention in diabetes, NCEP subtracts 30 points from the LDL-C goal of 130 to get to a goal of 100 mg/dL. I suggest that the LDL-C goal for secondary prevention in diabetes be lowered by 30 mg/dL to be less than 70. It seems appropriate to subtract 30 points for diabetes with and without atherosclerosis, and 20 points in primary and secondary prevention for patients with insulin resistance without diabetes. This is an unofficial suggestion, based on relative risk data, and on the fact that both patients with diabetes and those with insulin resistance are likely to have small dense LDL particles, which results in our doubly underestimating their risk for CHD.

STUDIES OF STATINS IN PATIENTS WITH DIABETES
OR INSULIN RESISTANCE

There is some evidence that statins might reduce the CHD risk in patients with diabetes or insulin resistance. Many studies of statins have included patients with diabetes, and on average, these patients have experienced roughly the same risk reduction as patients without diabetes. For instance, the Heart Protection Study (HPS), the largest statin-based study, showed that patients with diabetes had at least the same risk reduction as all other patients taking 40 mg of simvastatin daily.[6]

Patients with a baseline LDL cholesterol less than 100 mg/dL, those already at the goal level, still had the same event reductions as did those starting with an LDL cholesterol above the goal. There are two ways to interpret this finding. Perhaps LDL is irrelevant, and does not need to be measured; perhaps all patients should be taking statins regardless of their LDL levels. Another possibility is that LDL is still important but that the goals may be too conservative (too high). In either case, statins should probably be used in most high-risk primary prevention and secondary prevention patients.

LDL levels are still relevant, however. In sub-analysis of the HPS subjects, by tertile of baseline LDL cholesterol, the relationship between LDL-C levels and CHD events among patients receiving treatment continued to be linear well below an LDL-C of 100 mg/dL. Although these data do not prove that lowering an LDL of 130 to 70 would reduce CHD events correspondingly, they certainly strongly suggest that this is the case. Some large ongoing studies, in particular TNT (Treating to New Targets)[7] and SEARCH (Study of the Effectiveness of Reducing Cholesterol and Homocysteine),[8] will test formally the question whether lowering LDL levels with high or low doses of the same statin will provide further event reduction. However, I believe existing evidence is sufficient to justify setting an LDL cholesterol goal of 70 in especially high-risk patients.

In the recent ASCOT (Anglo-Scandinavian Cardiac Outcome Trials), atorvastatin was used in patients under treatment for hypertension.[9] Disappointingly, those with diabetes seemed not to have as much benefit as those without diabetes, and the same trend appeared for those with and without the metabolic syndrome. However, the results for these groups did not differ statistically. Additionally, the CARDS (Collaborative Atorvastatin Diabetes Study) using atorvastatins in type 2 diabetes was stopped early because the drug showed a benefit.[10] I believe this justifies the opinion that atorvastatin is effective in diabetes, as are the other statins.

In the LIPS (Lescol Intervention Prevention Study), fluvastatin or placebo was given to a large number of patients with or without diabetes shortly after an angioplasty. The response in patients with diabetes tended to be greater than that in those without.[11] Therefore, in most cases statin therapy should be continued, or started if necessary, after an angioplasty.

AFCAPS/TEXCAPS (Air Force/Texas Coronary Atherosclerosis Prevention Study), a primary prevention study using lovastatin, showed interesting results relevant to the metabolic syndrome.[12] Baseline HDL-C, an important component of the metabolic syndrome, was a strong inverse determinant of event reduction with therapy. Patients with HDL-C below 40 mg/dL had especially dramatic benefits. Interestingly, a similar pattern has been seen in other statin studies, among which is the 4S (Scandinavian Simvastatin Survival Study).[13] Those with both a low HDL and a high triglyceride tended to show much greater benefit with statin therapy. Although statins are not regarded as being very effective in raising low HDL levels or lowering high triglycerides, they appear effective in these cases.

HATS (HDL-Atherosclerosis Treatment Study) was a secondary prevention trial in which an antioxidant vitamin cocktail appeared somewhat harmful.[14] As you would expect, combining a statin with niacin produced lower LDL levels and higher HDL levels, especially among the larger HDL particles, and large decreases in Lp(a) and triglycerides. With regard to the angiographic endpoints, statin plus niacin completely prevented the disease progression seen in the placebo group, but adding antioxidants completely blocked this benefit. The same was true for clinical events. The mechanisms for this loss of effect are not established, but it is known that antioxidants can have pro-oxidant effects in certain settings. Owing to these findings, it would seem wise to suggest that patients taking antioxidant vitamins consider discontinuing them.

In addition, the event reduction seen with statin plus niacin is much greater than has ever been seen with statin monotherapy. Because this was a relatively small study, the results cannot be considered definitive, but other statin combination studies have shown similar findings. Combination therapy should have more consistent application in the highest-risk patients.

TRIALS OF FIBRATES FOR LIPID REDUCTION

In the Helsinki Heart Study, a primary prevention trial, fibrates plus niacin produced a large event reduction in patients with diabetes, perhaps even a little larger than in those without it. Most of the benefit with gemfibrozil was seen below a baseline HDL of about 42 mg/dL.[15]

In the VA-HIT (Veterans Affairs High-Density Lipoprotein Cholesterol Intervention Trial), a study of secondary prevention with gemfibrozil, there was no change in LDL cholesterol, but LDL particle size was increased and particle number decreased.[16] There was also a large decrease in triglyceride levels and a modest but significant increase in HDLs, which seemed to account for a significant reduction in CHD events. These effects were seen to a comparable degree in diabetes and in the metabolic syndrome without diabetes.

Perhaps the best predictor of event reduction was HDL levels during treatment. Those whose HDL-C rose over 35, with gemfibrozil, had very few events, while those whose HDL remained below 29 had many more events. Triglyceride levels during the trial, paradoxically, did not predict the event rate, despite the fact that the triglyceride change was much greater than the HDL change. Many have interpreted these data to say that the HDL increase with gemfibrozil accounts for the event reduction. but this is not definitive. These are post-hoc analyses and therefore only suggestive.

DAIS (Diabetes Atherosclerosis Intervention Study is the biggest study so far with fenofibrate, but its results were inconclusive. In patients with diabetes, angiographic progression of atherosclerosis was reduced and the reduction in coronary events was promising but not statistically significant.[17] Thus, evidence for clinical benefits with fenofibrate is weaker than for gemfibrozil. The ACCORD (Action to Control Cardiovascular Risk in Diabetes) study will provide further and perhaps more definitive data about the clinical effects of fenofibrate.[18]

Many believe that niacin is harmful for patients with diabetes and the metabolic syndrome, because it can worsen glycemic control, perhaps owing to an increase in insulin resistance. Despite this widespread perception, in the Coronary Drug Project, patients with diabetes and metabolic syndrome had at least as great, if not greater, clinical event reduction as did patients with normal glucose metabolism.[19] Therefore niacin, fibrates, or statins, alone or in combination, are effective in atheroprevention in patients with the metabolic syndrome or diabetes.

Recently the Coronary Drug Project data have also been analyzed for the effects of niacin on glycemic control and on other aspects of the metabolic syndrome.[20] The average patient in this study started out with borderline impaired fasting glucose. There was a slight increase in fasting glucose levels with niacin treatment, but it was only about 6%, and did not progress during the study. By the end of the trial, the placebo patients' glucose levels had increased to equal those of the niacin patients. Therefore the adverse effects of niacin are relatively trivial, and it can be on the list of usable drugs in metabolic syndrome and/or Type 2 diabetes.

Given the fact that we now have drugs that inhibit the absorption of cholesterol, we can assess the reciprocal relationship between cholesterol synthesis and cholesterol absorption. Both fasting serum insulin and, to a lesser degree, fasting blood glucose are positively related to cholesterol synthesis. This means that patients with insulin resistance or Type 2 diabetes are generally over-synthesizers of cholesterol. One reason why statins work well in insulin resistance is probably that they inhibit cholesterol synthesis.

Naturally, obesity is associated with an increase with cholesterol synthesis —about a 50% increase, compared with normal-weight patients. There is, however, a reciprocal drop in cholesterol absorption in obesity; the two tend to be inversely related. Weight loss, as one might expect, will tend to reduce cholesterol synthesis, and will therefore increase cholesterol absorption as measured by serum campesterol levels, which are markers of cholesterol absorption.

Investigators in Finland, as part of the 4-S trial, separated a small cohort of patients into quartiles of cholesterol absorption, as measured by campesterol levels. The hyper-absorbers were less heavy and had a lower body mass index (BMI), while hypo-absorbers had lower HDL-C levels and higher triglyceride levels.[21] Probably most of the hypo-absorbers had the metabolic syndrome. In this analysis, simvastatin reduced CHD events in those with low to average cholesterol absorption, but it did not reduce events in hyper-absorbers. As you might expect, the hyper-absorbers also did not show much LDL reduction with statin therapy. This could be interpreted to mean that there is a group of patients who should not be treated with statins. However, it is not yet justified to apply this result clinically. First, it has not yet been duplicated. Second, there is no clinically practical standardized test for cholesterol absorption or synthesis.

To summarize this point, we have two contrasting types of patients with regard to cholesterol metabolism. First, there are the high-synthesizer, low-absorption patients, who often have obesity, insulin resistance, and type 2 diabetes, and may be more likely to have the ApoE-2 phenotype. On the other side are the patients who are lean and insulin-sensitive, who may be more likely to have the ApoE-4 phenotype and be less responsive to statins. For such patients, it may be best to start treatment with a cholesterol-absorption inhibitor or another non-statin drug, perhaps niacin or fibrate. It is probably not correct to ask whether we should exclusively use statins or cholesterol absorption inhibitors in a given patient, however, because initial treatment with either one upregulates the other process and appears to make the other class of drugs more effective. More information is required before making firm clinical recommendations.

INFLAMMATION, ATHEROGENESIS, OBESITY
AND INSULIN RESISTANCE

Inflammation also appears important in atherogenesis, especially in patients with diabetes or insulin resistance, probably through several mechanisms. LDL itself is pro-inflammatory, and small dense LDLs is even more so. Low HDL-C, and high triglycerides, which usually coincide, also appear to be pro-inflammatory, although for unrelated reasons. Vascular endothelial dysfunction is also pro-inflammatory and pro-atherogenic. Healthy endothelium serves as a barrier to entry of atherogenic lipoproteins and inflammatory cells into the artery wall and is a major source of endogenous antioxidants. Also, because fat cells produce inflammatory cytokines, obesity is a pro-inflammatory state. C-reactive protein (CRP) is a strong marker, and perhaps even a mediator, of inflammation.

Excess sympathetic nervous activity, common in obesity and insulin resistance, may also play a role in inflammation. A prothrombotic state is important in its own right as a contributor to inflammation. Unfortunately, usable clinical measurements of thrombotic tendencies have proven difficult to develop.

LDL is pro-inflammatory and pro-atherogenic even if particles are large, and more so if they are small. In a pro-inflammatory state HDL, the so-called "good" lipoprotein inhibits many pro-inflammatory and pro-atherogenic processes, among them: (1) adhesion molecule expression by endothelium; (2) the resulting adhesion of inflammatory cells to endothelium; (3) the chemotaxis or movement of inflammatory cells across the endothelial barrier; and (4) the modification of LDL (which it may even be able to reverse). Also, and perhaps most importantly, HDL can promote cholesterol removal from inflammatory foam cells and perhaps from plaque in general. Thus, potentially, HDL can block every deleterious effect of LDLs. Raising HDL levels is an attractive therapeutic goal, but not enough is known about this to allow extensive official clinical guidelines.

There are other beneficial effects of HDL. It seems to block the actions of two key pro-inflammatory factors, TNF-α and NF-κB, thus halting what otherwise tends to be a downward inflammatory spiral.

C-reactive protein, a major marker of inflammation, is a good CHD risk predictor in itself. However, exactly how much it may enhance risk prediction in combination with conventional lipid factors is more controversial. C-reactive protein correlates strongly with the metabolic syndrome. Its levels rise almost 10-fold between people who have none of the five criteria for metabolic syndrome and those who have all five. In fact, C-reactive protein may be a quick and simple way of estimating whether someone has metabolic syndrome. Alternatively, if one does clinical screening for the metabolic syndrome as recommended in the ATP III guidelines, one may gain relatively little from a C-reactive protein level in cases where metabolic syndrome is clearly either ruled in or ruled out.

C-reactive protein levels fall with statin therapy, and a higher baseline level may predict greater benefit with statins. As is the case with metabolic syndrome, patients with high C-reactive protein levels seem to have a higher risk untreated and a greater risk reduction with various treatments, including statins and even aspirin. C-reactive protein levels may be a useful guide in cases where it is unclear whether or not therapy will be of benefit.

American Heart Association guidelines on the subject of CRP testing suggest its use in the same situations recommended above for extended lipid profiles. This situation is intermediate-risk primary prevention, when further information is needed to decide whether or not to prescribe lipid-lowering therapy for atheroprevention.

ESTROGEN REPLACEMENT AND LIPIDS

Estrogen raises C-reactive protein (CRP) levels. This would be expected to be pro-atherogenic, suggesting that estrogen replacement should be particularly harmful in the setting of a high baseline CRP. Interestingly, the opposite appears to be the case: The higher the baseline CRP, the greater the apparent benefit of estrogen replacement. Estrogen has many anti-inflammatory effects and probably, on balance, reduces inflammation rather than increasing it. Since CRP reflects the degree of inflammation, those individuals with more inflammation would be expected to have greater benefit from an anti-inflammatory agent. This is believed to be the case with statins and aspirin, for example. In my opinion, the increased levels in patients taking estrogen is simply a non-specific effect of oral estrogen, which is to increase hepatic synthesis of many proteins, including likely C-reactive protein, which is made mainly in the liver. Estrogen replacement also seems to help prevent the onset of diabetes and of atherosclerosis in the metabolic syndrome and diabetes.[22] Looking at this another way, CHD risk goes up with increasing baseline quintile of C-reactive protein level, but the excess risk is largely eliminated by estrogen treatment. This effect is reminiscent of what appears to happen to CHD risk in cases of low HDL-C and/or high triglycerides, treated or untreated with statins and fibrates.

What is the explanation for the increase in CHD events in the first year or so of estrogen treatment, seen in the HERS (Heart and Estrogen/Progestin Replacement Study)[23] and WHI (Womens' Health Initiative)[24] trials? Estrogen may well promote both the likelihood of rupture of pre-existing vulnerable plaques and the size of any rupture, because of its effect of increasing matrix metalloproteinase (MMP)-9 activity. Once a plaque is ruptured, the likelihood and extent of a subsequent CHD event is probably determined primarily by the size and extent of the resulting thrombosis. Estrogen is definitely pro-thrombotic. Thus, the effects of estrogen on CVD events should depend on whether one is giving it in the early stages of atherogenesis, where its effects should be favorable, or in the late stages, where its effects are likely harmful.

There may also be an independent effect of the time the body has experienced low postmenopausal levels of estrogen. This deficiency probably alters estrogen receptor activity, and if present long enough may reduce or even reverse the ability of estrogen to reduce atherosclerosis. Another possibility is that women who have hot flashes at the menopause are more likely to have favorable vascular effects by replacing estrogen. Any and all of these are reasonable explanations for the striking observation that estrogen started early in the menopause for vascular symptoms (as in routine clinical use and as in the observational trials) appears to greatly decrease CVD events, while estrogen started late in the menopause and with few or no preceding deficiency symptoms (as done rarely in clinical practice but as done in HERS and WHI) may increase CVD events, at least temporarily. Unfortunately, the official interpretation of HERS and WHI, that estrogen replacement must always be adverse or at best neutral for CVD risk, seems to be an overextrapolation of studies done in a clinically irrelevant setting.

When estrogen is initiated late in the menopause, and not for vascular symptoms (as was done in the WHI), negative consequences are likely. However, there is no evidence from the WHI that stopping estrogen after 5 years, as is now uniformly and strongly recommended, is in any way necessary or helpful.

Obesity and weight loss regulate many inflammatory markers. Their levels are increased in obesity, but in every case that excess is erased by losing weight. Weight loss not easy to achieve, but sustained weight loss can reverse the proinflammatory state of obesity. The same is true of endothelial function. Obese patients have impaired endothelial function, but with weight loss, function improves to that seen among normal-weight individuals.

In summary, the increase in risk for cardiovascular disease is high both for patients with diabetes and for those with metabolic syndrome, and the many mechanisms of this increase are similar (except for the hyperglycemia of diabetes). The basic treatment for both disorders is the same: target insulin resistance first, and then the dyslipidemias. The preferred agents are the same: statins, fibrates, and niacin, and potentially hormone replacement in postmenopausal women. Hormone treatment may help prevent the onset of Type 2 diabetes, and appears to reduce CHD risk more in patients with diabetes than among those without it.

REFERENCES

1. STAMLER, J., O. VACCARO, J.D. NEATON & D. WENTWORTH. 1993. Diabetes, other risk factors, and 12-yr cardiovascular mortality for men screened in the Multiple Risk Factor Intervention Trial. **16:** 434–444.
2. MCCARTNEY, P., H. KEEN & R. JARRETT. 1983. The Bedford Study: observations on retina and lens of subjects with impaired glucose tolerance and in controls with normal glucose tolerance. Diabetes Metab. **9:** 303–305.
3. EXPERT PANEL ON DETECTION, EVALUATION, AND TREATMENT OF HIGH BLOOD CHOLESTEROL IN ADULTS. 2001. Executive Summary of the Third Report of the National Cholesterol Education Program (NCEP) Expert Panel on Detection, Evaluation, and treatment of High Blood Cholesterol in Adults (Adult Treatment Panel III). JAMA **285:** 2486–2497.
4. THE HEART OUTCOMES PREVENTION EVALUATION STUDY INVESTIGATORS. 2000. Effects of an angiotensin-converting-enzyme inhibitor, ramipril, on cardiovascular events in high-risk patients. New Engl. J. Med. **342:** 145–153.
5. HAFFNER, S.M. *et al.* 1998. Mortality in coronary heart disease in subjects with type 2 diabetes and in non-diabetic subjects with and without prior myocardial infarction. New Engl. J. Med. **339:** 229–234.

6. HEART PROTECTION STUDY COLLABORATIVE GROUP. 2002. MRC/BHF Heart Protection Study of cholesterol lowering with simvastatin in 20,536 high-risk individuals: a randomised placebo-controlled trial. Lancet **360:** 7–22.
7. LAROSA, J.C. *et al.* 2005. Intensive lipid lowering with atorvastatin in patients with stable coronary disease. New Engl. J. Med. **352:** 1424–1435.
8. MCMAHON, M. *et al.* 2000. A pilot study with simvastatin and folic acid/vitamin B12 in preparation for the Study of the Effectiveness of Additional Reductions in Cholesterol and Homocysteine (SEARCH). Nutr. Metabl. Cardiovasc. Dis. **10:** 195–203.
9. PETER, S. *et al.* 2003. Prevention of coronary and stroke events with atorvastatin in hypertensive pateints who have average or lower-than-average cholesterol concentrations. Lancet **361:** 1149–1158,
10. COLHOUN, H.M. *et al.* 2004. Primary prevention of cardiovascular disease with atorvastatin in type 2 diabetes in the Collaborative Atorvastatin Diabetes Study (CARDS): multicentre randomised placebo-controlled trial. Lancet **364:** 685–696.
11. SERRUYS, P.W. *et al.* 2002. Fluvastatin for prevention of cardiac events following successful first percutaneous coronary intervention. A randomized controlled trial. JAMA **287:** 3215–3222.
12. DOWNS, J.R. *et al.* 1998. Primary prevention of acute coronary events with lovastatin in men and women with average cholesterol levels. JAMA **279:** 1615–1622.
13. SCANDINAVIAN SIMVASTATIN SURVIVAL STUDY GROUP. 1994. Randomised trial of cholesterol lowering in 4444 patients with coronary heart disease: The Scandinavian Simvastatin Survival Study. Lancet **344:** 1383–1389.
14. BROWN, B.G. *et al.* 2001. Simvastatin and niacin, antioxidant vitamins, or the combination for the prevention of coronary disease. New. Engl. J. Med. **345:** 1583–1595.
15. FRICK, M.H. *et al.* Helsinki Heart Study: Primary-prevention trial with gemfibrozil in middle-aged men with dyslipidemia. New Engl. J. Med. **317:** 1237–1245.
16. RUBINS, H.B. *et al.* 1999. Gemfibrozil for the secondary prevention of coronary heart disease in men with low levels of high-density lipoprotein cholesterol. New Engl. J. Med. **341:** 410–418.
17. DIABETES ATHEROSCLEROSIS INTERVENTION STUDY INVESTIGATORS. 2001. Effect of fenofibrate on progression of coronary-artery disease in type 2 diabetes: the Diabetes Atherosclerosis Intervention Study, a randomised study. Lancet **357:** 905–910.
18. See http://www.accordtrial.org.
19. THE CORONARY DRUG PROJECT RESEARCH GROUP. 1975. Clofibrate and niacin in coronary heart disease. JAMA **231:** 360–381.
20. CANNER, P.L. *et al.* 2005. Benefits of niacin by glycemic status in pateints with healed myocardial infarction (from the Coronary Drug Project). Am. J. Cardiol. **15:** 254–257.
21. MIETTINEN, T.A. *et al.* 1998. Baseline serum cholestanol as predictor of recurrent coronary events in subgroup of Scandinavian simvastatin survival study. Br. Med. J. **316:** 1127–1130.

22. KANAYA, A.M. *et al.* 2003. Glycemic effects of postmenopausal hormone therapy: The Heart and Estrogen/progestin Replacement Study: A randomized, double-blind, placebo-controlled trial. 2003. Ann. Intern. Med. **138:** 1–9.
23. HULLEY, S. *et al.* 1998. Randomized trial of estrogen plus progestin for secondary prevention of coronary heart disease in postmenopasual women. JAMA **280:** 605-613.
24. WRITING GROUP FOR THE WOMEN'S HEALTH INITIATIVE INVESTIGATORS. 2002. Risks and benefits of estrogen plus progestin in healthy postmenopausal women: Principal results from the Women's Health Initiative randomized controlled trial. JAMA **288:** 321–333.

Dietary Fat and Health: The Evidence and the Politics of Prevention

Careful Use of Dietary Fats Can Improve Life and Prevent Disease

WILLIAM E.M. LANDS

ABSTRACT: Every year, more young people start the slow progressive injury that eventually becomes cardiovascular disease and death. It could be prevented with nutrition education, but medical efforts focus more on treatments for older people than on preventing primary causes of disease in young people. Two avoidable risks are prevented by simple dietary interventions: (1) Eat more omega-3 and less omega-6 fats, so tissues have less intense n-6 eicosanoid action, and (2) eat less food per meal to lower vascular postprandial oxidant stress. An empirical diet–tissue relationship was developed and put into an interactive personalized software program to aid informed food choices.

KEYWORDS: essential fatty acids; omega-3; omega-6; polyunsaturated fatty acids (PUFAs); highly unsaturated fatty acids (HUFAs); eicosanoids; thrombosis; inflammation; atherosclerosis; prenylated proteins; platelet activating factor (PAF); oxidized LDL

Much of this chapter echoes talks given 10, 20 and 30 years ago,[1–3] presenting information which failed to percolate effectively into clinical practice or preventive nutrition. As a result, I continue trying to find different methods of effective education so that chronic diseases may be prevented in the elderly. Recent efforts involve two distance-learning web sites with useful "homework" for everyone who wants to learn. One site, for education about essential fatty acids[a] has many details to help people understand the effects of nutritionally essential fatty acids. The other[b] has been hosted by the Office of Dietary Supplements for almost four years, and was upgraded recently with additional background information on how diet affects eicosanoids and how eicosanoids affect health and life.

[a]http://efaeducation.nih.gov/
[b]http://ods.od.nih.gov/eicosanoids/
Address for correspondence: William E.M. Lands, Ph.D., 6100 Westchester Park Drive, Apt. 1219, College Park MD 20740 USA. Voice/fax: 301-345-4061.
wemlands@att.net

Ann. N.Y. Acad. Sci. 1055: 179–192 (2005). © 2005 New York Academy of Sciences.
doi: 10.1196/annals.1323.028

The death rate from heart attacks in the United States is among some of the worst in the world.[4] FIGURE 1 demonstrates that death, not life, begins at 40. That is the age at which people begin to lose colleagues and become aware of death. Students feel invulnerable, because not many 30-year-olds die. However, among my peers in their 70s, 1 or 2 per 100 are likely to die of ischemic heart disease in any year.[1] Clinicians say that arterial damage and calcium deposition is just a matter of aging, and that nothing can be done about that. I don't believe that a bit. In Japan, age-specific death rates for coronary heart disease are much lower.[5] However, an apparent inevitability about this is rooted in American lifestyles, all the way back to childhood.

FIGURE 1, presented in 1993,[1] has results added from the PDAY (Pathological Determinants of Atherosclerosis in Youth) study,[6-8] which documented this problem definitively. The problem became apparent 50 years ago, when young soldiers were being killed in Korea. Autopsies showed coronary artery damage in 20-year-old Americans, but not in native Koreans.[9]

Results from the PDAY study[6-8] show that effective primary prevention of atherosclerosis needs to begin with adolescents. FIGURE 1 suggests that by the time American men are 55 years old, most already have inflammatory

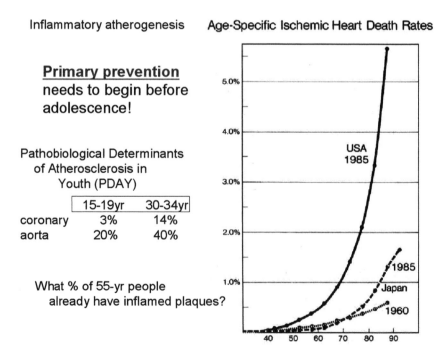

FIGURE 1. Inflammatory atherosclerosis begins developing before adolescence. (Presented in 1993;[1] results added from the PDAY study.[6-8]

plaques in their arteries. Intervention then is really secondary prevention.[10] The effective new technique of electron beam computerized tomography is maturing into a wonderful diagnostic tool.[11] Unfortunately, knowing that you have a lot of calcium in your arteries doesn't tell you how to get rid of it or how to prevent it from accumulating further. We still have a lot of biochemical work to perform.

Real primary prevention doesn't fit programs or goals of pharmaceutical companies, because they cannot make money by preventing the diseases they treat.[10] They work with treatment-oriented groups who aren't interested in educating people about specific dietary interventions that prevent causes of risk. One avoidable risk, an imbalance between intake and expenditure of energy, has received a lot of attention in the last two years. There is a need for further discussion about how it affects vascular inflammation and oxidant stress.

One solution is to eat foods that provide less energy per meal, as noted later in this chapter (FIG. 3). A second avoidable risk is the current severe imbalance between omega-3 and omega-6 nutrients. Most people are completely oblivious to it, but that imbalance is easily corrected by adjusting dietary intakes to more omega-3 and less omega-6 fats. The current imbalance in America is just a happenstance of food marketing.[12] Unfortunately, priorities of corporate health groups will favor the status quo over any action that prevents disease and suffering without adding to corporate profits.[10, 12]

FIGURE 2 shows the consequence of this imbalance. The horizontal axis shows that apparently healthy normal people around the world have different balances of omega 6 and omega 3 in their HUFAs (highly unsaturated fatty acids) because of the different foods they eat.[13,14] The HUFAs are pivotal in the body's healthy self-healing actions. Epidemiology shows that when HUFAs in the body are 70 or 80% omega 6, coronary heart disease rates are around 200 per 100,000.[4] In contrast, people in Spain or Italy have HUFAs containing about 60% omega 6 and 40% omega 3,[10] and their CHD mortality rate is around 120 per 100,000. In Japan, the traditional proportions of HUFAs are about 35–40% omega 6 and 60–65% omega 3, and the heart attack rate in Japan is about one-fourth to one-fifth that in the United States.[5] In Greenland, coronary heart disease is almost undetectable.

Many investigators do not like transnational epidemiology, claiming that genetic diversity impairs interpretation. However, genetic diversity within the United States is probably greater than the mean genetic difference between the United States and Japan. Now we have data from three groups in Quebec, within the same province of the same country on the same continent with the USA. There are urban Quebecois who eat foods that generate HUFA proportions similar to those of people in Chicago and Detroit and New York.[15] On the other hand, in villages north of Quebec City, there are Quebec Cree Indians with different ethnic food habits that give them a different HUFA pattern and mortality rate.[16] Further north in Quebec, Inuits have a lower average n-6

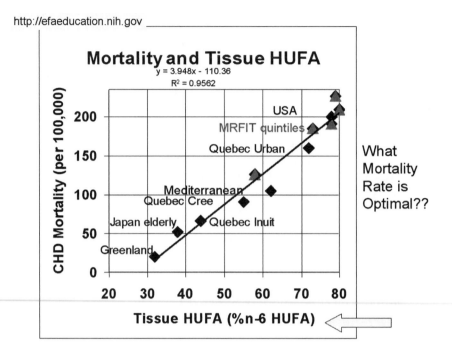

FIGURE 2. Coronary heart disease mortality is proportional to n-6 HUFA in plasma HUFA. Available at <http://efaeducation.nih.gov/sig/personal.html> .

HUFA composition and a lower mortality rate.[17] The trend is clear, even though the Inuit diet has changed tremendously during the last 40 years and is now far more heterogeneous. Indeed, dietary heterogeneity worldwide is the important variable for preventive intervention, more so than genetic variability. Environmental food variability is driving variability in CHD mortality.

Essential fatty acids are polyunsaturated fatty acids (PUFAs) required by all mammals. Like vitamins, these are not produced within the body, and must come from the diet. They are of two types, n-3 and n-6. Linoleic is a n-6 PUFA (18:2n-6) and alpha-linolenic is the n-3 PUFA (18:3n-3). When we eat those acids, our body converts them into longer chain-length, highly unsaturated fatty acids (HUFAs).[c]

What people eat in their diet determines the proportions of HUFAs in their tissue membrane phospholipids. In my first 15 years of academic life, I worked on lipid metabolism[18] and was highly cited on that topic. In 1964, when researchers in Stockholm reported that the n-6 HUFA, arachidonic

[c]http://efaeducation.nih.gov/sig/overviews.html

acid, was converted to the potent hormone, prostaglandin,[19] I hypothesized that HUFA for these hormones comes from the 2 position of the phospholipids in human tissues. But is HUFA converted to eicosanoids on the phospholipids and stored, or is it first hydrolyzed before the free hormone is synthesized? Collaborating with the researchers in Stockholm, I found that the HUFAs in phospholipids were hydrolyzed and then converted to eicosanoids. The hormone then acts at a receptor and generates a signal, which is usually a transient, reversible event that returns to basal state.[20,21]

By the late 1960s, we knew that omega-6 eicosanoids and omega-3 eicosanoids were involved in inflammatory processes. Later, I studied the mechanism by which fatty acid oxygenases act. This requires lipid hydroperoxide activators.[20] Eliminating the peroxides eliminates the ability to make a prostaglandin. Peroxides are also required to activate ribonucleotide reductase, and the free radical is essential to make deoxyribonucleotides for new DNA. The eicosanoids, and the peroxide tone that regulates them, are usually under tight control.[22]

For 15 years I studied aspirin-like non-steroidal anti-inflammatory drugs (NSAIDs),[23,24] working with drug companies to develop new patented drugs for treatment. During the 70s, dozens of eicosanoids were isolated.[21] Nearly all healthy human tissues use eicosanoid modulations of physiologic responses in a rapid transient manner.[20] However, uncontrolled excessive production of omega-6 eicosanoids over prolonged periods of time is associated with heart attacks, thrombotic stroke, arrhythmia, arthritis, asthma, headaches, dysmenorrhea (menstrual cramps), inflammation, tumor metastases and osteoporosis.[21,25] We had been looking at essential vitamin-like fatty acids as "angels" but in excessive amounts they turn into devils. When the body goes out of control, something must be done, and it became my goal to prevent this loss of control.

Two brief narrated presentations covering these general issues are available on the Internet.[d] The distance-learning site for the Office of Dietary Supplements has a section on dietary reference intakes[e] with a graph and citations.[f] These show that most people are eating on the order of 20 times more of the essential vitamin-like n-6 linoleic acid than they need. As with vitamin A and vitamin D, from which the body makes potent hormone-like compounds, there is a probable risk in excessive intakes. The website notes evidence for requiring these substances in amounts on the order of 0.5% of calories or less, but a day's menu in the United States far exceeds that.

To design an effective prevention strategy, one needs to identify causal mechanisms by asking how people die. From this point of view, the role of cholesterol[26, 27] has been portrayed in a misleading fashion for 25 years. Al-

[d]http://efaeducation.nih.gov/sig/beginners.html
[e]http://efaeducation.nih.gov/sig/dietary2.html
[f]http://efaeducation.nih.gov/sig/dri.html

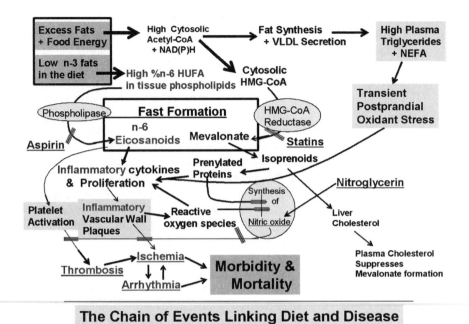

The Chain of Events Linking Diet and Disease

FIGURE 3. Two primary imbalances link diets to disease and death. Modified from an earlier figure[1] at <http://efaeducation.nih.gov/sig/dietdisease.html>.

though some lipoproteins may increase death, cholesterol itself was never proven to kill anyone. However, those who market anti-cholesterol drugs will never mention that fact. To consider primary prevention of heart attacks, we worked backward with the diet–disease concepts shown in FIGURE 3, by stating that a death from heart attack is a death from ischemia, which is exacerbated by arrhythmia, and from thrombosis, which was brought on by a predisposition to inflammatory plaques in the arteries. All three of these processes are exacerbated by n-6 eicosanoids (FIGURE 3). The release of inflammatory cytokines and cell proliferation are enhanced by omega-6 eicosanoids formed from dietary fats.

Inflammatory vascular wall plaques cause ischemia and stimulate thrombosis. Thrombosis is driven by thromboxane, one of the major eicosanoids discovered 29 years ago.[28] Thromboxane causes platelets to clump, causes calcium movement, and causes thrombosis. The omega-6 derivative (TX_{A2}) has the same effect; the omega 3 (TX_{A3}) also has that effect, but to a limited degree.

Aspirin, statins, and nitroglycerin are used widely to diminish the processes set in motion by the two nutritional imbalances shown in the upper left of FIGURE 3. In 1979, when I lectured[2] about these issues in Switzerland and the

Netherlands, the socialized medicine systems in those countries were paying for expensive coronary bypass surgery, and governments were considering preventive nutrition as an economic measure. However, proponents of medications and surgery were not interested in what they regarded as nutritional behavior modification. I scorned the clinicians' disinterest in nutrition at the time, but now I see they may be right. Often it is easier to persuade people to have surgery than to persuade them to change their ideas about what to eat.

What can we do to change people's behavior? Our responsibility is to inform people properly, and their responsibility is to learn what we are trying to teach. The two dietary interventions that people need to learn are shown in the upper left-hand corner of FIGURE 3. Eat more omega-3 and less omega-6 fats to have less-intense n-6 eicosanoid actions. Also, eat less high-energy food per meal to cut transient postprandial oxidant stress three times a day, a thousand times a year. Even when it's 99.9% reversible, the remaining one-tenth of a percent creates another irreversible inflammatory locus every year. By the time people are in their 70s, and the postprandial stress has excess n-6 HUFA and pro-inflammatory eicosanoids, then their condition is seen to move downward in FIGURE 3 and upward in FIGURE 1.

Low-density lipoprotein (LDL) and its phospholipids have some effect on events in FIGURE 3. When inflammatory sites oxidize those phospholipids, they create a platelet activating factor (PAF) agonist that binds the PAF receptor, causing calcium influx plus a stronger inflammatory response. That process has been understood, published, and well accepted for a decade. PAF and PAF mimics are potent calcium ionophores and inflammatory agents in mammalian tissue.[10] Electron beam computerized tomography, described in this volume by Dr. Harvey Hecht,[11] gives a good measure of atherosclerosis by measuring calcium accumulation. We need to learn more about what causes calcium to accumulate and how to prevent it and reverse the effect. Like LDL, high-density lipoprotein (HDL) is an aggregation of proteins, some of which are anti-inflammatory enzymes that destroy PAF and the oxidized phospholipid, preventing them from causing calcium entry and inflammation.[10]

Membrane phospholipids are limited in abundance, and the HUFAs compete for the limited space. If you eat a lot of n-6 fat, it displaces n-3 HUFAs and enhances n-6 eicosanoid formation (FIG. 3). If you eat a lot of n-3 fat, it displaces n-6 HUFAs. The enzymes are promiscuous and don't discriminate much between n-3 and n-6 HUFAs, which means that what you eat can change your body tissue.[13,14]

In the mid-80s, after a Nobel Prize had been awarded for discovery of eicosanoids and their physiology and I had done years of research on lipid metabolism and on NSAID mechanisms, it was well-know that n-6 thromboxane caused heart attacks and n-6 prostaglandins caused inflammation.[25] Pfizer gave me a grant to study the relationship between dietary n-6 and n-3 fats and the proportions of n-6 HUFA in body tissues. I developed and published an empirical predictive equation.[13,29]

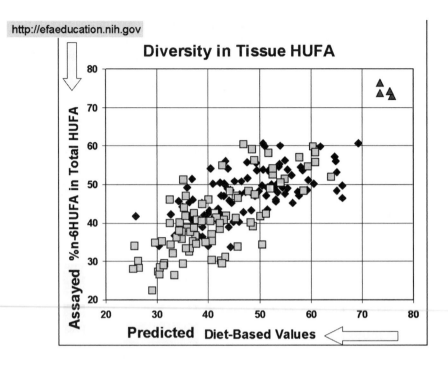

FIGURE 4. Predicted proportions of HUFA fit observed proportions. Previously presented[5] in 2003.

Sadly, I don't think many people read those papers, and I don't think anyone used the equation.[g] I then put it into a spreadsheet so people are not required to do any algebra. They can simply put numbers into a table and let the spreadsheet calculate the likely outcome.[h] FIGURE 4 shows that the equation predicts outcome with a correlation coefficient greater than 0.95. Dietitians carefully monitored the food that people ate, and that information inserted into the equation predicted values of the percentage of n-6 HUFAs in the total HUFA value. There is a good fit between predicted HUFA proportions and those observed by gas chromatographic analysis.[5]

The vertical scatter may be due to proteomics and genomics, whereas horizontal scatter is likely due to imprecise interviews. The group of people represented in the upper right hand in FIGURE 4 were 35-year-old Chicago women. The diamonds represent a group of 45-year-old dietitians in the cities of Japan, and the squares show 55-year-old rural Japanese men. They are all healthy people eating what they choose. The mean value for all people in ei-

[g]http://efaeducation.nih.gov/sig/hufacalc.html
[h]http://efaeducation.nih.gov/sig/dietbalance.html

ther FIGURE 4 or FIGURE 1 would not reveal much about any individual value or the risk of any individual in the group. Those who ate more dietary n-6 as linoleic acid (of which Americans eat a lot) acquired predictably higher proportions of n-6 HUFAs.[13,30]

I used the Pfizer grant to develop a diet–tissue relationship because people doing clinical interventions were making ineffective changes in the diet, too little and too late. Now you can sit down and plan effectively with a little "pocket calculator" at the learning site.[j] The outcome depends on four kinds of dietary essential fatty acid: the 18 carbon n-3 and n-6 and the long-chain n-3 and n-6 HUFA. Diet–tissue calculations can now be handled in a simple spreadsheet, using no algebra or arithmetic.

To illustrate the diet–tissue relationship, the family of curves in FIGURE 5 indicate how different mixtures of n-6 linoleate and n-3 HUFA in daily food create tissue HUFA proportions. Four different ethnic groups are shown as ovals. We still have a long way to go from the HUFA status for average Americans (200 deaths per 100,000 people) to where we might like to be. One cannot choose one's parents or one's genetics, but one can choose the food one puts in one's mouth.[30] It's a simple intervention for someone who is properly informed.

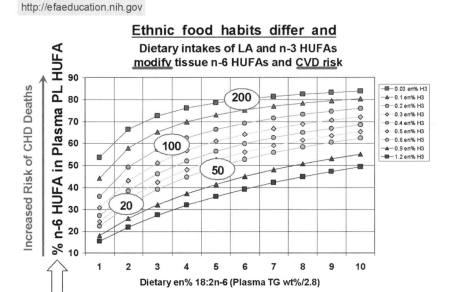

FIGURE 5. Diet–tissue relationship predicts the tissue proportions of n-6 HUFA in tissue HUFA. Available at <http://efaeducation.nih.gov/sig/food2.html>.

[j]http://efaeducation.nih.gov/sig/dietbalance.html

The HUFA proportions for 3,000 Quebec residents ranged from 15 to 91% n-6 HUFA. From FIGURE 2, people can choose their comfort level: what HUFA value they would like to have, and what heart attack risk they would accept. Many people don't want to choose; they want to be told the optimum value. FIGURE 2 makes it obvious that there is no optimum. As you go to higher proportions of n-6 HUFA, the risk grows worse.

Others can see the relationship and risk, but they want to be told which foods are best to eat. Although the distance-learning sites provide a great deal of background information, I decided to use the USDA data base of 6,000 different foods, more than 12,000 servings of food, to create an interactive, computerized, personalized, daily menu-planning program that can be downloaded free.[k] The program allows users to choose foods they want to eat, and it keeps the data managed to let them see whether the daily totals meet their personal goals of cardiovascular risk. The food software takes lifestyle information and tells users what their recommended daily energy allowance is (a value that most sedentary Americans exceed).[31] It also gives some background concepts of risk, and then asks users to choose their risk level and begin choosing foods. Once they look at specific foods, they can begin to see where the omega 6 is entering their diet. For example, the software tells users that the USDA describes a serving of applesauce as having 583 milligrams of 18-carbon omega-6 and only 48 milligrams of omega-3 with no long-chain HUFAs. You can't find any food that doesn't have quite a few milligrams of n-6 linoleate. People producing foods put in n-6-rich oils and raise the level even higher; some breads and muffins have huge amounts. The interactive software shows details and gives the bottom line—total daily total calories and the likely surrogate outcome of HUFA proportions. It also gives a few other dietary facts that dietitians are concerned about and want to convey.

What people really need to know is that their caloric intake is correct and their proportions of eicosanoid precursors are where they want them to be. The nature of a mealtime is that people eat more than they need at that moment and then have transient excess. That excess and its transient postprandial oxidant stress is the beginning of a problem.

If people ate only one meal a day, they would have a large bolus of carbons and electrons entering metabolic pathways. The liver would to make free radicals (and also make cholesterol) and the endothelial cells would respond with oxidant stress due to that postprandial bolus. If people ate smaller meals, five times a day, they would have smaller and more reversible oxidant stress; it would be still lower, with more n-3 and less n-6 HUFAs in the tissues. To take in less energy per meal, people should eat several small meals or snacks if they want. One of the underlying rules is to eat no more than you need.

The top predicted causes of death and disability[32] worldwide for 2020 (ischemic heart disease and unipolar major depression), and three top causes

[k]http://efaeducation.nih.gov/sig/kim.html

in developed regions (ischemic heart disease, cerebrovascular disease, and unipolar major depression) all seem linked to imbalanced omega-3 and omega-6 actions in tissues. We knew about n-6 eicosanoid mechanisms for thrombosis and inflammation 25 to 30 years ago. In the past five years, increasing evidence suggests that major depression, post-partum depression, and behavior disorders also relate to imbalances in omega-3 and omega-6 dietary intakes. Additional evidence showed important actions of n-3 HUFAs in brain function,[33] and the American Heart Association recently urged putting more n-3 HUFAs into daily diets.[34] The growing awareness of the importance of balancing n-3 and n-6 fats is evident from the single major personal health change recommended recently by the health and nutrition division members of the American Oil Chemists' Society: to eat more fish and take an omega-3 supplement.[35] Also, their most frequent advice to other people was to eat more seafood and fish.

In this volume, Dr. Richard Cutler[36] has given us a philosophical view of these issues. We tend to simplify matters that are complex. We use words like "gene" or "the genome" or "inflammation" or "aging," as if these phenomena were a single entity when, in fact, they are a mass of ill-defined parts. On the other hand, some things that are actually simple seem complex. FIGURE 3 outlines the chain of events that lead from food choices to morbidity and mortality. Three types of medication (aspirin, nitroglycerin, and statins) are noted, to show the step in the process at which these familiar drugs intervene. However, when we recognize the initial imbalances in our nutrition that cause cardiovascular death, we can design more effective primary prevention and better nutrition education for the public.

Inflammation was always important in vascular disease, and it was driven by excessive n-6 eicosanoid actions amplifying results of excessive food energy, producing more carbon and electrons than the body could deal with at any given moment. That led to increased cytosolic acetyl-CoA and HMG-CoA, which led to more mevalonate and prenylated proteins (FIG. 3) which are having effects that we didn't recognize 20 years ago. Some prenylated proteins block synthesis of nitric oxide and enhance inflammation. They come about because HMG-CoA reductase is pushed into making more mevalonate than necessary. We knew 25 years ago that plasma cholesterol gave negative feedback that suppressed cholesterol biosynthesis. We subsequently learned that plasma cholesterol suppresses the proteolysis of sterol regulatory element-binding protein, slowing activation of genes expressing fat-forming enzymes. The misimpression that cholesterol (a marker of excessive HMG-CoA reductase action) has been killing people, when the killers are actually vascular inflammation, thrombosis and arrhythmia, is one of the tragedies of biomedical science.[26,27]

The discussion in FIGURE 3 notes that lipoprotein (LDL) has phospholipids that form highly potent inflammatory agents on oxidation, regardless of cholesterol. Phospholipids in the LDL may be deadly. HDL may have cholesterol (and it has phospholipids), but it has enzymes that neutralize inflammatory oxidized phospholipid PAF mimics and PAF.[37] So HDL is beneficial and LDL is harmful, but it's absurd to talk about "bad cholesterol" and "good cholesterol." We can hope that the tragic detour that delayed understanding of nutritional causes and preventive interventions is nearly over, and that the organizations that could provide the necessary information will do so. Then a new day will dawn for the young people in whom every successive year perpetuates the slow progressive injury that leads to cardiovascular disease and death.

REFERENCES

1. LANDS, W.E.M. 1993. Eicosanoids and health. Ann. N.Y. Acad. Sci. **676**: 46–59.
2. LANDS, W.E.M., B. PITT & B.R. CULP. 1980. Recent concepts on platelet function and dietary lipids in coronary thrombosis, vasospasm and angina. Herz **5**: 34–41.
3. LANDS, W.E.M., P.R LETELLIER, L.H. ROME, et al. 1973. Inhibition of prostaglandin biosynthesis. Adv. Biosci. **9**: 15–27.
4. LANDS, W.E.M. 2003. Diets could prevent many diseases. Lipids **18**: 317–321.
5. LANDS, W.E.M. 2003. Functional foods in primary prevention or nutraceuticals in secondary prevention? Curr. Top. Nutraceutical Res. **1**: 113–120.
6. PDAY RESEARCH GROUP. 1990. Relationship of atherosclerosis in young men to serum lipoprotein cholesterol concentrations and smoking. A preliminary report from the Pathobiological Determinants of Atherosclerosis in Youth (PDAY) Research Group. JAMA **264**: 3018–3024.
7. MCGILL, H.C., JR., C.A. MCMAHAN, A.W. ZIESKE, et al. 2000. Associations of coronary heart disease risk factors with the intermediate lesion of atherosclerosis in youth. The Pathobiological Determinants of Atherosclerosis in Youth (PDAY) Research Group. Arterioscler. Thromb. Vasc. Biol. **20**: 1998–2004.
8. ZIESKE, A.W., G.T. MALCOLM & J.P. STRONG. 2002. Natural history and risk factors of atherosclerosis in children and youth: the PDAY study. Pediatr. Pathol. Mol. Med. **21**: 213–237.
9. ENOS, W.F., R.H. HOLMES & J. BEYER. 1953. Coronary disease among United States soldiers killed in action in Korea. JAMA **152**: 1090–1093.
10. LANDS, W.E.M. 2003. Primary prevention in cardiovascular disease: Moving out of the shadows of the truth about death. Nutrition, Metabolism and Cardiovascular Diseases **13**: 154–164.
11. HECHT, H.S. 2004. Cardiovascular risk assessment. Ann. N.Y. Acad. Sci. **1055**:this volume.
12. NESTLE, M. 2002. Food Politics: How the Food Industry Influences Nutrition and Health. University of California Press, Berkeley, CA.
13. LANDS, W.E.M., B. LIBELT, A. MORRIS, et al. 1992. Maintenance of lower proportions of n-6 eicosanoid precursors in phospholipids of human plasma in response to added dietary n-3 fatty acids. Biochem. Biophys. Acta **1180**: 147–162.

14. LANDS, W.E.M. 1995. Long-term fat intake and biomarkers. Am. J. Clin. Nutr. **61**(Suppl): 721S–725S.
15. DEWAILLY, E., C. BLANCHET, S. GINGRAS, et al. 2001. Relations between n-3 fatty acid status and cardiovascular disease risk factors among Quebecers. Am. J. Clin. Nutr. **74**: 603–611.
16. DEWAILLY, E., C. BLANCHET, S. GINGRAS, et al. 2002. Cardiovascular disease risk factors and n-3 fatty acid status in the adult population of James Bay Cree. Am. J. Clin. Nutr. **76**: 85–92.
17. DEWAILLY, E., C. BLANCHET, S. LEMIEUX, et al. 2001. n-3 Fatty acids and cardiovascular disease risk factors among the Inuit of Nunavik. Am. J. Clin. Nutr. **74**: 464–473.
18. LANDS, W.E.M. 1965. Lipid metabolism. Ann. Rev. Biochem. **34**: 313–346.
19. BERGSTROEM, S, H. DANIELSSON, D. KLENBERG et al. 1964. The enzymatic conversion of essential fatty acids into prostaglandins. J. Biol. Chem. **239**: PC4006–4008.
20. LANDS, W.E.M. 1979. The biosynthesis and metabolism of prostaglandins. Ann. Rev. Physiol. **41**: 633–652.
21. SAMUELSSON, B. 1979. Prostaglandins, thromboxanes, and leukotrienes: formation and biological roles. Harvey Lect. **75**: 1–40.
22. KULMACZ, R.J. & W.E.M. LANDS. 1997. Peroxide tone in eicosanoid signaling. *In* Oxidative Stress and Signal Transduction. H.J. Forman & E. Cadenas, Eds.: 134–156. Chapman & Hall. New York.
23. ROME, L.H. & W.E.M. LANDS. 1975. Structural requirements for time-dependent inhibition of prostaglandin biosynthesis by anti-inflammatory drugs. Proc. Natl. Acad. Sci. USA **72**: 4863–4865.
24. HANEL, A.M. & W.E.M. LANDS. 1982. Modification of antiinflammatory drug effectiveness by ambient lipid peroxides. Biochem. Pharmacol. **31**: 3307–3311.
25. LANDS, W.E.M. 1986. Fish and Human Health, Academic Press. Orlando, FL.
26. MOORE, T.J. 1989. Heart Failure. Simon & Schuster. New York.
27. RAVNSKOV, U. 2000. The Cholesterol Myths. New Trends Publishing, Inc. Washington, DC.
28. HAMBERG, M., J. SVENSSON & B. SAMUELSSON. 1975. Thromboxanes: a new group of biologically active compounds derived from prostaglandin endoperoxides. Proc. Natl. Acad. Sci. USA **72**: 2994–2998.
29. LANDS, W.E.M., A.J. MORRIS & B. LIBELT. 1990. Quantitative effects of dietary polyunsaturated fats on the composition of fatty acids in rat tissues. Lipids **25**: 505–516.
30. LANDS, W.E.M. 1991. Biosynthesis of prostaglandins. Annu. Rev. Nutrition **11**: 41–60.
31. Recommended Dietary Allowances, 10th Edition. 1989. National Academy Press, Washington, DC.
32. MURRAY, C.J.L. & A.D. LOPEZ. 1997. Alternative projections of mortality and disability by cause 1990–2020: global burden of disease study. Lancet **349**: 1498–1504.
33. SALEM, N., JR., B. LITMAN, H.Y. KIM et al. 2001. Mechanisms of action of docosahexaenoic acid in the nervous system. Lipids **36**: 945–959.
34. KRIS-ETHERTON, P.M., W.S. HARRIS & L.J. APPEL. 2002. Fish consumption, fish oil, omega-3 fatty acids, and cardiovascular disease. Circulation **106**: 2747–2757.

35. What the experts eat: the Health & Nutrition Division weighs in with nutrition advice. 2003. Inform (American Oil Chemists' Society) **14:** 116-117.
36. CUTLER, R.G. 2005. Oxidative stress profiling. Part 1. Its potential importance in the optimization of human health. Ann. NY Acad. Sci. **1055:** 93–135.
37. MARATHE, G.K., G.A. ZIMMERMAN & T.M. MCINTYRE. 2003. Platelet-activating factor acetylhydrolase, and not paraoxonase-1, is the oxidized phospholipid hydrolase of high density lipoprotein particles. J. Biol. Chem. **278:** 3937–3947.

Physical Activity and Aging

KERRY J. STEWART

Department of Medicine, Division of Cardiology, Johns Hopkins Bayview Medical Center, Johns Hopkins University School of Medicine, Baltimore, Maryland 21224, USA

ABSTRACT: **Most human beings experience peak physical performance in their late teens and begin a slow decline in their early 20s, whose course is greatly affected by the activity levels undertaken by individuals in the years that follow. Many studies provide evidence that in developed nations such as the U.S., a sedentary lifestyle contributes significantly to development of the major risk factors for age-related disease, prominent among them obesity, diabetes, and hypertension. Conversely, numerous studies document the benefits of physical activity, and in particular structured exercise programs, not only for reducing disease risk and improving physical performance, but also for enhancing substantially the quality of daily life. Aerobic and resistance training have complementary benefits, and can be undertaken at almost any age and physical condition, given appropriate medical clearance and supervision as warranted.**

KEYWORDS: **aging; physical activity; physical fitness; exercise; diseases af aging; cardiovascular disease, Alzheimer's disease; activities of daily living; body mass; obesity; muscle mass; quality of life**

FITNESS AND AGING: A TWO-WAY STREET

FIGURE 1 is a modification of a graphic that is commonly presented at an aging conference. It leads the audience through some of the pathways by which aging leads to disease. The arrows in the original graphic pointed one way, with increased fatigueability, muscle weakness, decreased endurance capacity, muscle wasting, all leading to decreased physical activity, and then eventually, through other pathways, to diseases such as heart disease. The modification is that some of the arrows now point in both directions. The justification for this modification is the considerable evidence that physical inactivity contributes to many of the adverse changes that occur with aging.

Address for correspondence: Kerry J. Stewart, Ed.D,, Professor of Medicine, Johns Hopkins Bayview Medical Center, 4940 Eastern Avenue, Baltimore, MD 21224. Voice: 410-550-0870; fax: 410-550-7727.

kstewart@jhmi.edu

Ann. N.Y. Acad. Sci. 1055: 193–206 (2005). © 2005 New York Academy of Sciences.
doi: 10.1196/annals.1323.029

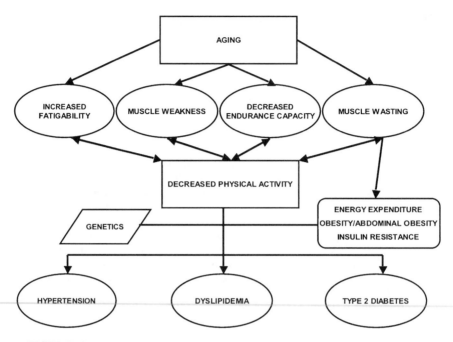

FIGURE 1. A commonly presented figure showing selected pathways by which changes upon aging lead to disease, All of the arrows in the original figure pointed one way, with increased fatigueability, muscle weakness, decreased endurance capacity, and muscle wasting leading to decreased physical activity, and eventually to disease. The *arrows in the middle* have been modified to point in both directions, indicating that physical activity itself (independent of aging) causes increased fatigueability, muscle weakness, decreased endurance capacity, and muscle wasting.

Physical inactivity speeds up the aging process in many people, whereas increased physical activity slows it down in others.

The typical aging curve suggests that most physiological functions improve from birth through the late teens. Most of these functions commonly level off in the mid-20s and then it's generally downhill from there for most physical and cognitive functions. However, the rate of change is not equal among individuals. What is clear is that there are several modifiable mediating factors on the aging curve. Among the key modifiable factors are physical activity, nutrition, body fat, muscle mass, and smoking, each of which can either delay or accelerate the aging process.

Our current understanding of the relationship between lifestyle and disease risk is not particularly new. In the recent biography of Benjamin Franklin by Walter Isaacson,[1] there is a story that demonstrates Dr. Franklin's understanding of the effects of activity and nutrition on health. In his later years, he suffered from gout and kidney stones. In his unique story-telling style,

Franklin says to The Gout, which is portrayed as a person, "What have I done to merit these cruel sufferings?" The Gout answers, "Many things. You have eaten and drank too freely, and you have much indulged those legs of yours in their indolence." "Who is [it] that accuses me?" asks Franklin. "It is I, even the gout." And Franklin responds, "What? My enemy in person? For you would not only torment my body to death, but ruin my good name, reproach me as a glutton and a tippler? Now all the world that knows me will allow that I'm neither the one nor the other." The Gout responds, "The world may think as it pleases, but I very well know that the quantity of meat and drink proper for a man who takes a reasonable degree of exercise would be too much for another who never takes any." In many ways, Dr. Franklin understood the notion of preventive medicine and healthy living, although, like many people today, he did not follow his own advice.

SEDENTARY LIFESTYLE: A FEW REALITIES

The sedentary lifestyle is a major contributor to the leading causes of death among adults in the United States.[2] It has been estimated that about 15% of the 1.6 million chronic health conditions that are newly diagnosed each year are due to a sedentary lifestyle alone, independent of other risk factors.[3] Unfortunately, according to the American Heart Association Biostatistical Fact Sheet for 2002 (FIG. 2),[4] about 30% of the American population performs no exercise at all. About 40% or so does some exercise, whereas only about 27%

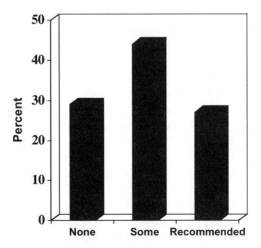

FIGURE 2. The number of adults in the U.S. who meet recommended guidelines for physical activity. (Adapted from the American Heart Association Biostatistical Fact Sheet for 2002.)

of the adult population engages in exercise at the recommended levels that would provide protection against the chronic diseases that occur in aging. The problem of physical inactivity is not only limited to older people but also exists across all age groups. The relative risk of coronary disease associated with physical inactivity, depending on the study, ranges anywhere from 1.5 to 2.5. This risk is comparable to that of high blood cholesterol, hypertension, and cigarette smoking.

The increasing problem of type 2 diabetes may also be related to physical inactivity. Among persons 70–75 years of age, approximately 25% have type 2 diabetes.[5] It is estimated that as many as 25% of all nursing-home residents have diabetes,[6,7] and they tend to be younger than other patients in the nursing home because diabetes accelerates the aging process. The prevalence of diabetes increased to almost 8% in 2001 from 7.3% in the previous year, or an overall increase of about 8%.[8] This increased risk of diabetes is closely linked to the increasing prevalence of overweight and obesity. For example, the prevalence of obesity, defined as a body mass index (BMI) greater than 30 kg/m,[2] which is the threshold for the category of obesity, was 21% higher in 2000 compared to the previous year.

In the Nurses Health Study,[9] each hour a day spent walking reduced both the risk of developing obesity and diabetes. The reduction in risk is about 25% for obesity and about 35% for diabetes. However, every two hours of daily television watching, or every increase of 2 hours a day, increases the risk. It is noteworthy that the risk was greater from watching television than from being inactive in other sedentary activities such as sitting or driving. Though further research is needed to explain this finding, it might be that when people watch television, they are often eating. It is also noteworthy that the risk for developing diabetes and obesity related to inactivity is independent of other types of activity that the individual does during the day. Even at higher levels of physical activity, for both men and women, the risk of type 2 diabetes and obesity each increase with more television watching.

Though obesity is a problem in older people, it starts in youth, and by middle age, many individuals are overweight or obese. The observation that obesity at a younger age affects health in the senior years is illustrated by the results of the Chicago Heart Association Detection Project.[10] This project followed about 6,700 men and women, aged 36 to 64 at baseline, who had completed a 26-year follow-up by the time they were 65 years or older. The relationships of the baseline BMI, characterized as either normal weight, overweight or obese, to the 26 year follow-up data for various measures of health status were examined. It was found that lifting and carrying groceries, climbing flights of steps or walking several blocks were more difficult among both men and women who were obese when they were younger.

It is important to understand the distinction between the terms "physical fitness" and "physical activity." The key features of each of these separate constructs are listed in TABLE 1. Some studies measure physical fitness

TABLE 1. Physical fitness versus physical activity

Physical Fitness

Measured as capacity to perform or sustain physical work

Measured as performance such as time to complete an event or lift a weight

Measured as a physiological variable such as maximal oxygen uptake or heart rate response

Physical Activity

Measured as habitual patterns of energy expenditure during work or leisure time activities or tasks

Measured by self-report or interview surveys, direct observations, or electronic monitoring devices

TABLE 2. Health-related versus performance-related components of physical fitness

Health-Related Fitness

Cardiorespiratory endurance: Ability to provide oxygen to muscles

Muscle strength: Ability to exert force during a single effort

Muscle endurance: Ability to execute repeated contractions over time

Flexibility: Ability to move through a range of motion

Body composition: % body fat, central vs. peripheral obesity

Performance-Related Fitness

Speed

Agility

Balance

Coordination

whereas others measure physical activity, so it is important to keep these differences in mind when evaluating research findings.

Fitness also falls into two major categories—one related to health and the other to the ability to perform a task or sport. The key characteristics of health and performance-related fitness are shown in TABLE 2. These components of fitness have important distinction. Though speed and agility are needed to play sports, like tennis or golf, *skill* in sports is not a predictor or measure of health.

BENEFITS OF FITNESS FOR AGING ADULTS

In 1998, the American College of Sports Medicine published a statement on exercise and activity for older adults.[11] It concluded that exercise reduces and prevents a number of functional declines in aging. Some of the key points are as follows: Older individuals at any age can generally adapt and respond

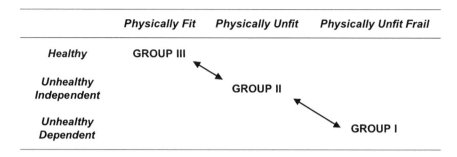

FIGURE 3. World Health Organization health-fitness gradient. Most older adults fall along this continuum, with good health at one end, and physical frailty at the other. Exercise can improve health and fitness status, whereas a lack of exercise will accelerate its decline.

to both endurance and strength training. Aerobic or endurance training maintains and improves cardiovascular function, whereas strength training helps offset the loss in muscle mass and strength associated with normal aging. Regular exercise also results in improvements in bone health, a reduction of risk of osteoporosis, improvement in postural stability, and increases in flexibility. These factors lead to a reduced risk of falls, a major cause of morbidity and mortality in the elderly. Exercise provides many psychological benefits including preserved cognition, alleviation of depressive symptoms and behavior, and an enhanced sense of self-efficacy, the concept of personal control. Individuals feel that they are in charge of their health when they are active. And increased physical activity certainly contributes to a healthy, independent lifestyle with improvements in functional capacity and quality of life.

The World Health Organization (WHO) has presented a health and fitness gradient for categorizing the functional status of older persons (FIG. 3).[12] Most older adults fall somewhere on this continuum. Persons in group 3 are physically fit and healthy; those in group 2 are physically unfit and unhealthy, but still independent, while individuals in group 1 are physically unfit, frail, unhealthy, and dependent on others. What is noteworthy is that individuals can move either up or down this continuum. A key benefit of exercise is that it may enable some older individuals to regain their independence and restore their health, at least to some degree

The WHO guidelines[12] also outlined some of the benefits of physical activity that fall into three broad categories: physiological, psychological, and social. Some physiological benefits are immediate, such as improvement in glucose, catecholamine levels, and improved sleep. The longer-term benefits of physical activity include improvement in aerobic or cardiovascular endurance, muscle strengthening, flexibility, balance, and velocity of movement, which is a critical factor in the definition of frailty.

Immediate psychological benefits include relaxation, reduction of stress and anxiety, and enhanced mood state. The longer-term effects are improvements in some of these quality-of-life measures plus improvements in cognitive ability, motor control, and skill acquisition. These latter benefits would allow older persons to continue to play golf and tennis and other activities they might enjoy. There are also several social benefits that accrue from being active. An important immediate benefit of physical activity is to empower older people to gain a sense of control over what they do and increased involvement in social and cultural activities. One such benefit is "enhanced intergenerational activity," where the older person can play tennis, golf, or go on a ski trip with children or even grandchildren.

Numerous studies support the American College of Sports Medicine's recommendations that older persons stay active. For example, the Honolulu Heart Program followed about 2,600 older men, aged 71 to 93, for 2 to 4 years.[13] During follow-up, 109 of the men developed clinical coronary disease. After adjustment for age and the traditional cardiovascular disease risk factors, men who walked less than 0.25 miles a day had twice the risk of having a clinical cardiac event, than those who walked 1.5 miles a day (FIG. 4). Among those who walked 0.25 to 1.5 miles a day, there was some benefit, but their risk was still considerably higher than that among those who were able to walk even more. These are important health benefits that could be derived simply by encouraging elderly persons to walk more. Though skeptics will always note that this is a cross-sectional study and that the individuals who walked more were healthier at baseline, cross-sectional and randomized stud-

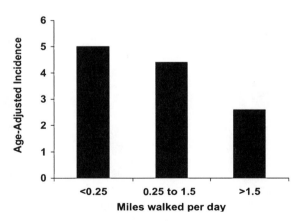

FIGURE 4. Walking and coronary heart disease in elderly men in the Honolulu Heart Program. Men who walked <0.25 mile/day had twice the risk of CHD as those who walked >1.5 mile/day (5.1% versus 2.5%; P <0.01). Men who walked 0.25 to 1.5 mile/day were also at a higher risk than men who walked longer distances (4.5% versus 2.5%; P < 0. 05).

ies alike consistently suggest that physical activity is a building block for good health.

Muscle strength and muscle mass play a significant role in the ability to function on a day-to-day basis, as well as the ability to participate in recreational activities. There is a well-defined decline in muscle mass with age, which is known as sarcopenia.[14,15] In the mid-20s, the loss is about a 4% per decade. By the mid-50s it accelerates markedly to where the loss is about 10% of muscle mass per decade. Most commonly, the loss of muscle tissue is accompanied by an increase in fat tissue. Thus, body composition shifts as an individual ages. Although an older individual may maintain the same body weight over many years, it is most likely that his or her percentage of body fat has increased, while the percent of lean body tissue has decreased.

What therapies are available for reversing sarcopenia, reducing fat, and increasing muscle strength? Some studies have demonstrated that the use of growth hormone and sex steroids will increase lean tissue and reduce fat mass.[16] However, these treatments are often associated with serious adverse side effects. Some animal studies have demonstrated that gene therapy may increase muscle mass. Gene therapy has hope for the future, yet little is available today for humans. One proven option is "gym" therapy. It is widely available, produces many desired physiological outcomes, and has few side effects.

To examine the effects of resistance training, 84 healthy adults, 60 to 83 years old, were randomly assigned to a low-intensity exercise program, a high-intensity exercise program, or a control group.[17] They exercised 3 times

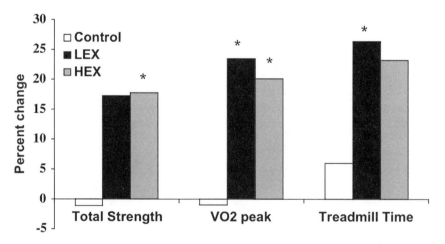

FIGURE 5. Six months of resistance exercise in elderly men and women. * $P < 0.05$ from control group. LEX = low-intensity exercise; HEX = high-intensity exercise. Both exercise groups experienced improvements in muscle strength and cardiovascular endurance capacity.

a week for 6 months, performing 12 resistance exercises each session on weight machines. The low-intensity group exercised at 50% of one repetition-maximum, performing one set. The high-intensity group worked out at 80% of one repetition-maximum. (One repetition maximun refers to the maximal amount of weight that can be lifted one time during strength testing.) After 6 months, in both genders, there were marked improvements in total strength in both intensity groups. Though subjects were doing resistance training, they also reached higher levels of maximal oxygen uptake on a treadmill, and markedly increased treadmill times (FIG. 5). The increases in aerobic capacity and treadmill time were moderately correlated with several measures of leg strength, with Pearson R values ranging from 0.4 to 0.54. There were no substantial differences between the low- and high-intensity resistance groups, suggesting that aerobic endurance is possibly limited by muscle strength. Individuals who lack the muscle strength to walk on the treadmill may not reach the true limits of their maximal aerobic capacity. Resistance training, therefore, may also contribute to increases in aerobic capacity by allowing individuals to reach higher levels of work.

Another study examined the development of disability in a large cohort of elderly men and women who were members of a running club.[18] They were compared to age-matched, community-based individuals who were of comparable health but were not runners. They were followed for 13 years. Among the runners, for both genders, there was a very low increase in their disability scores, compared to those who were not exercisers on a regular basis. Even after adjustment for age, the results were essentially the same. There was a rise in disabilities among the runners in their 80s, so they were not protected forever. But there was a clear-cut advantage among runners in terms of living more years with a lower level of disability or delay in disability compared to controls.

The prevention of disabilities for activities of daily living (ADL) was studied in older persons with osteoarthritis of the knee.[19] Participants were 250 individuals, 60 years or older, who had radiographic evidence of arthritis in the knee, but were free of ADL disabilities at baseline. They were randomly assigned to 18 months of aerobic or resistance exercise, or to an attention control group. The exercise program consisted of 3 months of supervised exercise, followed by a 15-month home-based program. The ADL items consisted of bathing, eating, and dressing. After 18 months, there was a higher risk of developing ADL disability in the controls compared with the exercisers.The greater preservation of ability to perform ADLs was similar in the aerobic and resistance exercise groups.

A recent study[20] evaluated a program of exercise plus behavior management in 153 community-dwelling patients with Alzheimer's disease who were enrolled in a program called Reducing Disability in Alzheimer's Disease or RDAD. It was a 3-month home-based exercise program, including training of a caregiver. Controls received usual care. The exercise program included aerobic, strength, balance, and flexibility exercises. Among the key results, at 3 months, was that more of the patients in the RDAD group exercised at least 60 minutes a week. They also reported fewer days of restricted physical activity and their SF-36 scores for physical role functioning improved at 3 months. After 2 years, they were still better than the routine care group, suggesting that exercise coupled with behavior interventions may have a role in maintaining some degree of function and improvement of quality of life in people with this disease.

Another health issue relevant to older persons is body composition. Obesity is associated with insulin resistance, glucose intolerance, diabetes, hypertension, and coronary disease. Abdominal obesity, the fat around the waist and within the abdominal cavity, may be a critical risk factor for developing these metabolic and cardiovascular diseases. Although abdominal visceral fat is not seen except by MRI or CT imaging, it is believed to be more harmful than other kinds of fat. Reduced abdominal fat is an important feature of the exercise training response and may help to improve cardiovascular health, particularly in reducing the risks of type 2 diabetes and hypertension.

FIGURE 6 shows the results of a study we recently completed (unpublished observations). Men and women, 55 years and older, were randomized to a 6-month exercise program, consisting of aerobic and resistance training. The reduction in abdominal visceral fat is in the range of 22%. At the same time, the change in body weight on the scale was about 2 kilograms. These results suggest that abdominal visceral fat is reduced by exercise training, indepen-

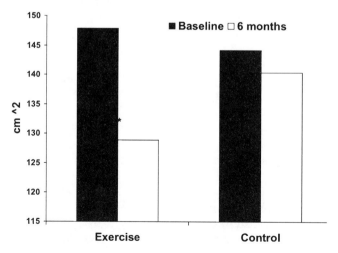

FIGURE 6. Abdominal visceral fat with 6 months of exercise training in older hypertensive men and women (unpublished observations). The reduction in abdominal visceral fat is in the range of 22%. The change in body weight was about 2 kilograms. $N = 34$ exercisers; $N = 35$ controls. * $P < 0.001$ for the change from baseline.

dent of changes in total body weight. Patients may get discouraged if they are not losing body weight, yet it is likely that they have improved their health because of a reduction in visceral fat.

HOW MUCH EXERCISE, AND WHAT KIND, IS OPTIMAL?

The general recommendation for exercise is that every U.S. adult should accumulate 30 minutes or more of moderate-intensity physical activity on most, and preferably all, days of the week.[21] The 30 minutes of moderate activity can be done either all at once, but those people who are unlikely to put aside the time to do 30 minutes all at once should at least accumulate 30 minutes of activity over the course of the day.

There are also recommendations for a structured exercise program for older adults. These are 3 to 5 times per week, for 30 to 45 minutes, at an intensity that is vigorous enough to raise the pulse rate to 70–80% of the maximal heart rate.[22] Older persons may require longer warm-up periods and longer cool-down periods as their cardiovascular systems adjust to the work and adjust back to the resting state. It is fairly common, in older people, to get a pooling of blood in the legs when they stop exercising suddenly. This can lead to a drop in blood pressure, and often people feel dizzy. If individuals do a long cool down, perhaps 10 to 15 minutes, and gradually taper off exercise, symptoms can be avoided.

The American Heart Association has recommended resistance training for individuals with or without cardiovascular disease.[23] For healthy individuals, the AHA recommends a moderate level at 50% of maximal effort, performing 8 to 10 exercises, 2 to 3 times a week. Persons with cardiovascular disease will eventually get up to this level but they should start at a lower intensity, in the range of 30 to 40% of maximal effort. Our research has shown in selected patients that it is safe to start weightlifting 2 to 3 weeks after myocardial infarction.[24] Patients who have undergone coronary artery bypass surgery should wait about 6 weeks before starting upper-body resistance training, not because of the heart but because time is needed for healing of the sternum. Patients with coronary disease are started at one set of 10 to 15 repetitions. They lift 10 to 15 times, 2 to 3 times a week. Over a course of 2 to 3 months, those with heart disease essentially follow the same exercise prescription, resistance training, as those without heart disease.

The American College of Sports Medicine says that most adults do not need medical consultation before starting a moderate-intensity program.[22] However, those individuals who have been inactive, men over 40, women over 50, and those who have multiple risk factors should see a physician before starting a vigorous program. For these individuals, an exercise stress test is usually warranted, and they should be warned that if they develop symptoms with moderate exercise they must stop and see the doctor. Persons with known disease and other complications should be examined and given the appropriate advice. Nevertheless, most individuals can start at least a moderate-level program without the need for extensive medical testing.

KEY FEATURES OF AEROBIC AND RESISTANCE TRAINING

Aerobic exercise, which includes activities like jogging, walking, swimming, and cycling, increases heart rate and breathing for extended periods of time. Resistance training is the contraction of muscle done against a force. The classic example is weightlifting, although for many older individuals who either do not have access to weight machines or for whom the lowest weight on a machine is too heavy, hand weights, bar bells, dumb bells, and stretching bands are excellent alternatives. Resistance training increases muscle strength and endurance and increases lean body tissue.

Aerobic and resistance training each promote benefits in the health-related fitness factors which were described earlier. The estimated weightings in terms of physiological benefits, however, are often substantially different. Aerobic exercise is more likely to produce increases in maximal oxygen uptake and stroke volume, maximal exercise times, reduction in heart rate and blood pressure at rest and during submaximal exercise, and to burn more calories than resistance training. It also contributes more to reductions in percent of body fat. Resistance training, conversely, has a greater impact on muscle strength and endurance, although these improvements often lead to improvements in aerobic performance in older persons if muscle capacity at baseline is a limiting factor. With resistance training there are benefits on lean body mass and prevention of frailty and falls in older people. For both forms of exercise similar benefits accrue in terms of improvement in bone mineral density, glucose tolerance, insulin sensitivity, and body weight. Although aerobic exercise burns more calories, resistance training increases lean body mass, which will increase basal metabolism.

In summary, let's turn again to the conversation between Dr. Benjamin Franklin and his adversary.[1]

> FRANKLIN: It's not fair to say I take no exercise. What I do very often, going out to dine and returning in my carriage.

> GOUT: Flatter yourself no longer that half an hour's airing in your carriage deserves the name of exercise. Providence has appointed few to roll in carriages while he has given to all a pair of legs, which are machines infinitely more commodious and serviceable. Be grateful then, and make a proper use of yours. Observe when you walk that all your weight is alternately thrown from one leg to another, thus accelerating the circulation of the blood. The heat produced in any given time depends on the degree of this acceleration. The fluids are shaken. The humor is attenuated and the secretions are facilitated. All goes well. The cheeks are ruddy and health is established.

REFERENCES

1. ISAACSON, W. 2003. Benjamin Franklin: An American Life. Simon and Schuster. New York.
2. BOOTH, F.W. *et al.* 2002. Waging war on physical inactivity: using modern molecular ammunition against an ancient enemy. J. Appl. Physiol. **93:** 3–30.
3. F.W. BOOTH & M.V. CHAKRAVARTHY. 2002. Cost and Consequences of Sedentary Living: New Battleground for an Old Enemy. 2002. President's Council of Physical Fitness and Sports Research Digest, Series 3, No. 16. President's Council on Physical Fitness and Sports. Washington, D C.
4. Heart Disease and Stroke Statistics: 2002 Update. Heart Disease and Stroke Statistics.
5. FRANSE, L.V. *et al.* 2001. Type 2 diabetes in older well-functioning people: who is undiagnosed? Data from the Health, Aging, and Body Composition study. Diabetes Care **24:** 2065–2070.
6. SINCLAIR, A.J. *et al.* 2001. Prevalence of diabetes in care home residents. Diabetes Care **24:** 1066–1068.
7. HAUNER, H. *et al.* 2001. Undiagnosed diabetes mellitus and metabolic control assessed by HbA(1c) among residents of nursing homes. Exp. Clin. Endocrinol. Diabetes **109:** 326–329.
8. MOKDAD, A.H. *et al.* 2003. Prevalence of obesity, diabetes, and obesity-related health risk factors, 2001. JAMA **289:** 76–79.
9. HU, F.B. *et al.* 2003. Television watching and other sedentary behaviors in relation to risk of obesity and type 2 diabetes mellitus in women. JAMA **289:** 1785–1791.
10. DAVIGLUS, M.L. *et al.* 2003. Body mass index in middle age and health-related quality of life in older age: the Chicago Heart Association Detection Project in industry study. Arch. Intern. Med. **163:** 2448–2455.
11. AMERICAN COLLEGE OF SPORTS MEDICINE. 1998. ACSM Position Stand. Exercise and physical activity for older adults. Med. Sci. Sports Exerc. **30:** 992–1008.
12. CHODZKO-ZAJKO, W.J. 1997. The World Health Organization Issues Guidelines For Promoting Physical Activity Among Older Persons. J. Aging Phys. Activ. **5:** 1–8.
13. HAKIM, A.A. *et al.* 1999. Effects of walking on coronary heart disease in elderly men: the Honolulu Heart Program. Circulation **100:** 9–13.
14. DOHERTY, T.J. 2003. Invited review: aging and sarcopenia. J. Appl. Physiol. **95:** 1717–1727.
15. EVANS, W.J. & D. CYR-CAMPBELL. 1997. Nutrition, exercise, and healthy aging. J. Am. Diet. Assoc. **97:** 632–638.
16. BLACKMAN, M.R. *et al.* 2002. Growth hormone and sex steroid administration in healthy aged women and men: a randomized controlled trial. JAMA **288:** 2282–2292.
17. VINCENT, K.R. *et al.* 2002. Improved cardiorespiratory endurance following 6 months of resistance exercise in elderly men and women. Arch. Intern. Med. **162:** 673–678.
18. WANG, B. *et al.* 2002. Postponed development of disability in elderly runners: a 13-year longitudinal study. Arch. Intern. Med. **162:** 2285–2294.

19. PENNINX, B.W. *et al.* 2001. Physical exercise and the prevention of disability in activities of daily living in older persons with osteoarthritis. Arch. Intern. Med. **161:** 2309–2316.
20. TERI, L. *et al.* 2003. Exercise plus behavioral management in patients with Alzheimer disease: a randomized controlled trial. JAMA **290:** 2015–2022.
21. PATE, R. *et al.* 1995. Physical activity and public health. A recommendation from the Centers for Disease Control and Prevention and the American College of Sports Medicine JAMA **273:** 402–407.
22. ACSM's Guidelines for Exercise Testing and Prescription. 2000. Lippincott, Williams, and Wilkins. Baltimore, MD.
23. POLLOCK, M.L. *et al.* 2000. AHA Science Advisory. Resistance exercise in individuals with and without cardiovascular disease: benefits, rationale, safety, and prescription: An advisory from the Committee on Exercise, Rehabilitation, and Prevention, Council on Clinical Cardiology, American Heart Association; Position paper endorsed by the American College of Sports Medicine. Circulation **101:** 828–833.
24. STEWART, K.J, *et al.* 1998. Safety and efficacy of weight training soon after acute myocardial infarction. J. Cardiopulm. Rehabil. **18:** 37–44.

Would Doubling the Human Lifespan Be a Net Positive or Negative for Us, Either as Individuals or as a Society?

Point–Counterpoint

GREGORY B. STOCK[a] AND DANIEL CALLAHAN[b]

[a]Program on Medicine, Technology and Society, School of Public Health, University of California at Los Angeles, Los Angeles, California 90024, USA

[b]The Hastings Center, Garrison 10524, New York, USA

ABSTRACT: There is a significant possibility that over the next few decades science will make discoveries of a kind that might allow the doubling of the average human life span, from roughly 76 years now to 150. This development would, for many, represent the realization of a dream: that of enabling people to live much longer lives than at present, holding back death, which has often been seen as an ancient, unbeatable enemy. It would also raise a large number of unprecedented individual and social problems: Would we really want to live to 150? Is such a goal ethical? What would this putative longevity do to our present social structures and arrangements? Would we get a better society or a worse one?

KEYWORDS: longevity; lifespan; vitality; death; healthcare costs; life expectancy; population growth

POINT—EXTENDING OUR VITAL YEARS WOULD BE DESIRABLE FOR OUR SOCIETY

STOCK: The question before is us whether doubling human life span, and presumably adult life expectancies as well, would be beneficial for us as in-

Addresses for correspondence: Gregory B. Stock, Ph.D., Director, Program on Medicine, Technology, and Society, UCLA School of Public Health, 760 Westwood Boulevard, Los Angeles, CA 90024. Voive: 310-825-9715; fax: 423-487-7512.

gstock@signumbiosciences.com

Daniel Callahan, Director, International Program, The Hastings Center, Garrison 10524, NY. Voice: 914-424-4040.

callahand@thehastingscenter.org

This article has been modified and reprinted by permission from the *Journal of Gerontology: Biological Sciences* (2004) **59A**: 554–559.

Ann. N.Y. Acad. Sci. 1055: 207–218 (2005). © 2005 New York Academy of Sciences.
doi: 10.1196/annals.1323.030

dividuals or as a society. Those who believe such a development will arrive during the next generation or so are almost certainly overly optimistic, but we will examine here not that issue, but whether the goal itself is worthwhile, because the answer has significant public policy implications. Some critics of biotechnology have argued that such a development would be undesirable and that we should therefore discourage research to achieve the insights that might allow us to meaningfully intervene in the aging process.

It may seem self-evident that extending our vital years would be desirable, but so many people have argued the contrary that it is worth looking closely at both the personal and social consequences of such a development. I will argue that the benefits would not only be personal, but social as well.

On the personal side, life's larger trajectory, when looked at from afar, is a brutal one. If we live long enough, everything we love is eventually taken from us: our family, our friends, our health, our connections to the world around us—smell, taste, vision, hearing—our vitality, even our minds. Anyone who views the trajectory from youth towards decrepitude as idyllic should sit in a nursing home and contemplate a photo of the early years of someone who has become hunched and frail, or who is barely present at all. Who would not feel some sorrow at this diminution?

We've developed many ways of trying to accept these ravages, and death itself for that matter. The first strategy is to ignore this descent into ill health and death: We can simply pretend it isn't happening. This works when we're young, but becomes ever less effective as the years march by and our strength seeps from us. The second way is to deny death's finality: We can assert that the soul is eternal, that our memory will live on, that we are young at heart, that we are not older but better. A third way is to battle the process like Ponce de Leon did by slogging through Florida to discover the Fountain of Youth, like Dorian Grey, or like those engaged in anti-aging research because, in the backs of their minds, they hope to extend their own futures. Or we can accept this descent as sad but inevitable, and say that it's natural and can't be avoided, or even tell ourselves that it's the best thing and claim, like Leon Kass, the Chair of the President's Bioethics Advisory Commission, that death gives meaning to life.

Dan Callahan, I suspect, is smack dab in the middle of this last category, not only accepting aging, but in some ways, extolling its virtue and ultimate wisdom. I, on the other hand, see it as a sorry state of affairs. Frankly, I don't see how you can applaud our current life expectancies and rue their extension while truly saying "Yes" to life, unless you think we live in a perfect world, where everything happens to be optimal just as it is. And that idea of optimal design is hardly one you hear expressed with regards to any of the body's other frailties.

On the other hand, we alter the world around us all the time. We build and dam and plough. We domesticate animals and plants. We breed our pets to suit our personalities. If we accept that the proper trajectory is a "natural" life span, then we are accepting that more healthy life is not a general good for us, at least as individuals. This would seem to imply that less healthy life should perhaps be our goal. And if we were to accept that, a lot of changes are implied, the least of which is that we should terminate much of our public health effort and biomedical research.

Sure, at some point in our journey toward decrepitude, life can become so painful that it is difficult to bear, and the prospects ahead so grim that death can look like a rescuer. That is why we don't always mourn when we see an older person die—death is an escape from the woes of aging and disease. But the game of anti-aging medicine is to buy more youthfulness, not more decrepitude. If life shifts at some point from being a positive to being a negative, it does so not at some particular age, but as a result of the internal changes and debilities that accompany the process of life itself. And it stands to reason that delaying the arrival of those changes would delay this shift and add life that is of value to us individually. The cost of intervention might be too high, of course, but theoretically the personal cost could be brought down to very near zero, as is the case, say, for antibiotics that insulate us from infectious disease.

In my view, it is only at the point at which a person ceases valuing life itself that he or she would not see freely choose anti-aging interventions as being of personal benefit. To reject such an intervention for oneself is one's prerogative, but to try to deny it to others should not be. What about social costs, though? The global costs of more youth and vitality might be so high as to demand that individuals forego the obvious personal benefits of extended longevity.

Before we answer that question, let's think about how best to measure costs or benefits. The only metric that makes sense is personal. Life extension is of value if individuals value it, and if individuals value it a great deal, it is very valuable. Moreover, in our culture, people do value extended vitality and youth, because they strive for even its appearance, spending substantial sums on vitamins, cosmetics, and anti-aging medications that accomplish little or nothing. Without this broad desire for extended youth, there would not be so many charlatans and hucksters exploiting this quest. So, if actual anti-aging interventions come into being, we will forego them only in the face of very serious social costs.

In looking at the social costs of anti-aging medicine, we should consider interventions that are freely available and easily accessible not only because these would be the most challenging socially, but also because it is so easy to distort the distribution of even a great good and worry about issues of equity and justice that have little to do with the nature of the good itself. To try to weigh costs and benefits, I could list the advantages I see in doubling the span of our vital healthy lives. For example, such an intervention would give us a chance to recover from our mistakes, lead us towards longer-term thinking, and reduce healthcare costs by delaying the onset of the expensive diseases of aging. It would also raise productivity by adding to our prime years. It takes a long time to acquire the knowledge and experience to operate effectively in the increasingly complex world we live in, and just as we achieve this we begin to slow down. So, adding to our prime years would be of tremendous benefit now, just as it has been in the past. Yale economist William Nordhous, for example, claims that the dramatic increase in human life expectancy since 1900 has been responsible for about half the increase in our standard of living in the United States since then.

I could wave my hands and assert that these sorts of benefits outweigh the various social challenges that would come from changed patterns of wealth transfer, changed family dynamics, the unanticipated consequences of reduced intergenerational turnover, and the need for people to come up with new life plans that encompass these unprecedented extra decades. I could minimize the challenges of getting rid of dictators and even the aging tenured professors that academics always seem to worry about. I could assert that change always brings challenges and that our projections about the impact of something as monumental as doubling the human life span and adult life expectancies tell us more about our own values and beliefs than they tell us about what would really happen. I could insist that Dan Callahan had better have some very clear and dire social dangers in mind, if he wants to use their avoidance as justification for sacrificing decades of life for so many who value it deeply.

But the real issue is not how we weigh the debits and credits we see, but how we judge what to call a debit or a credit. As I see it, the value of a development to society at large is ultimately the sum of the value it generates for each individual in that society. Thus, if on average we benefit as individuals, then society will enjoy a net benefit. In some situations, of course, the supposed individual benefits are a mirage. The so-called *Tragedy of the Commons*, for example, occurs when apparent individual benefit evaporates or is short-lived if pursued by everyone. This happens when the supply of what is sought is limited so that everyone can't possibly have it, or when something that is sought is valued primarily because it shifts one's relative status in society and thus is no longer of value when possessed by all.

Anti-aging medicine is afflicted by neither of these attributes. In fact, the more aggressively it is pursued by more people, the more likely it is to arrive more rapidly and to end up being cheaper and more readily available to more people, even those who did not pursue it in the first place. In addition, the greater the number of people enjoying extended longevity, the more we ourselves would enjoy it. Many people claim that they don't want to live a longer life because they'd grow increasingly isolated as their friends and family aged and passed away. So, the access of others to such a medical intervention would increase, not decrease, its value to us. The circle is virtuous.

The public policy implication of this is that we should not only allow anti-aging research, but we should also pursue it aggressively to gain both the individual and the social benefits that would accrue. And if we believe that eventual success is likely—whether in decades, generations, or centuries—spending healthcare resources in its pursuit is a gift to future generations because such effort makes it more likely that they will be among the first to enjoy these benefits, rather than among the last—as we may be—to miss them.

I will go even further. To spend resources on our current health care needs, instead of on these future possibilities, is highly suspect if to do so we incur, as is now the case, deficits that will have to be paid by future generations. To sum up, anti-aging interventions are clearly of value to many individuals. Anti-aging interventions are advantageous to society as measured by the very assessment of its members. And as a consequence, we should be virtually compelled to pursue anti-aging medicine as aggressively as we possibly can.

COUNTERPOINT—SOCIETY WOULD GAIN NOTHING BY DOUBLING HUMAN LIFE EXPECTANCY

CALLAHAN: One of the advantages of getting older, and pursuing these issues, is that I now have more time to argue with people I think are quite wrong about this. I will try to show you why I think Dr. Stock is travelling down the wrong road. I am 73 years old and and spend a lot of time with people my age and older, which brings a certain amount of perspective to the question. I observe the trajectories of their lives to see how they are turning out. The average life expectancy has been greatly increased, particularly for those over 65 and it's continuing to increase. So we have before our eyes some of the *results* of extended life spans. We can observe what happens to people who are still in good health and still vigorous, and we can see how their lives turn out and how satisfied they are with their life. This is kind of a "natural experiment" with my own life and that of my peers.

I begin by suggesting four different models of longevity and give you a notion of the one that I think makes the most sense. One I will call *the natural progress model*; by that I mean that we continue doing what we are now doing—that is, trying to understand and improve the aging process. I'm not against anti-aging research. I'm in favor of improving the quality of research and the quality of aging research and the quality of the life of the elderly, but not deliberately trying to extend life. Whatever extension comes as a result of trying to improve quality we should simply regard as a by-product. One demographer has said that there has been an average gain of about 3 months a year for 160 years now in average life expectancy, and I suspect that will continue to go on. That's perfectly fine and that will come about by improving the social and economic living conditions of people, by better preventive care, and by better clinical medicine in later years. That's one model.

The second I call *the normalizing model*: We could work hard to reduce premature death, and aim to cluster everyone around the age of 85, which is the age Japanese women now reach, on average. If we got everyone clustered closer to the average of 85, this would be a pretty decent life, a life long enough to do most of the things you can do in life.

A third model is *the optimalizing model*: There was the famous French woman, Jeanne Calment, who lived to be 122. We could try to get everybody clustered around that age. We know that such a long life is biologically possible. It has happened. And there are, of course, more people these days living to 105, 110, 114, that that is not a crazy goal either.

Finally, there is *the maximizing model*, which is to attempting to double life expectancy.

I believe in the natural progress model. I think we are doing fine now. People are living longer, and improvements are continually being made. Life will be better for the elderly in the future, but I see nothing whatever to be gained by deliberately attempting to double life expectancy. My stance is very much a social stance. It seems to me irrelevant that a lot of people would like it. A lot of people like a lot of things that are bad for the collective good of the rest of us. The fact that many of us want to live longer says nothing about (*a*) whether it will be good for us as individuals to live much longer, and (*b*) whether this will result in a better society. We already have plenty of evidence of bad results stemming from people trying to pursue their individual welfare. It is hard to credit the argument, as Dr. Stock does, that if everybody gets what they want individually, we will collectively be better off. That is a great fallacy—reminiscent of Adam Smith's "invisible hand' argument—that we will get a good society by satisfying everybody's individual desires. That is a false notion of the way society and our collective lives work.

Let me raise three basic problems that have to be addressed if we are going to talk about radically extending life:

First, consider all of our present problems in the world, in our national and global community—problems of war, poverty, environment, job creation, social and familial violence, for instance. Are there any of those problems that would be solved by everyone's living a much longer life? I don't think so. I can't imagine it's going to help the environment very much. It's certainly not going to deal automatically with social and family violence, and it will not do away with the problems of war, poverty, and violence. One question then is to ask, "Will doubling our life span solve any of our current problems?" I can't think of one.

Secondly, what *new* social benefits would a much longer life expectancy confer on our society? Dr. Stock romanticizes about these new possibilities. Maybe it will happen, maybe it won't; who knows? Anybody can have sweet and lovely dreams about the future. But we have to ask the much tougher questions, and not just speculate, not assume we'll find ways to adjust, and that it will all turn out beautifully. We don't know that at all. Will we get new wisdom? One of the advantages of getting to being my age, and living with people my age, is that I realize that people my age do not have any greater wisdom. If we have greater wisdom, then I'm right and Dr. Stock, my junior, is wrong. I haven't gotten any wiser between 50 and 73. I was probably wiser at 50 than I am now. And most of the people I live with who are my age or older don't seem to be a bit wiser. If I want to talk about interesting things, I look for vitality and drive: I go to young people. One bit of advice my mother gave me in her old age was "Cultivate young friends. Don't hang around people who are old." She was absolutely right about that.

Do I see new energy? I live around some people who are very sick. But mainly I live among the affluent elderly between the ages of 70 and 95. They are in good health, they have money, and they can take nice cruises or just putter about. They go to Scottsdale and play golf. But they don't seem to have any new energy, and they don't have any new serious agendas. How many people at this meeting are over 70? Not many. All of us over 70 know how rare it is to find many of "our kind" at meetings, looking at new things. Most of the older people have dropped out. I doubt that if you give most people longer lives, even in better health, they are going to find new opportunities and make new initiatives. Maybe they will want to play more rounds of golf, but they generally aren't going to come up with a lot of brand new ideas.

But the hardest question is how we should restructure society to deal with persons who live to a very old age. That question has to be looked at realistically. We know it would change the structure of job opportunities and of job mobility. We know it would change the ratio of young and old, and if you are going to examine the question of extending life expectancy, you are going to have to look at the whole problem of child bearing and child rearing. Those two go together. What's going to happen to these issues in such a society? Leaving aside questions of equitable distribution, if we have very different ideas about living much longer lives, how are we going to design a social security system? What will we do with Medicare where people have different desires for different lengths of time? A lot of people these days are in pretty good health because of expensive drugs and the like. Is Medicare going to support that indefinitely? I think we will have a lot of problems.

It is not enough to speculate idealistically about the benefits without speculating equally about the potential downside. Each one of the problems I mentioned has to be solved in advance. The dumbest thing for us to do would be to wander into this new world and say, "We'll deal with the problems as they come along." I don't think that would work. A doubling of life expectancy would fundamentally change society. If this could ever happen, then we'd better ask what kind of society we want to get. We had better not go anywhere near it until we have figured those problems out.

The problem can't be solved by looking at what individuals might like. I suggested at the beginning that what individuals like is not a good predictor of what is going to be good for society. I would also mention, from my own life experience, that I don't see any correlation between length of life and satisfaction with life. Certainly, one doesn't want to die prematurely, but beyond that, it seems to me that living a decent life—assuming one hasn't died as a child, or in middle-age as an adult—really has nothing to do with the *length* of life. It's how you live your life and the kind of goals you set for yourself that determine the ultimate value of life. The length by iteself is not a fundamental value.

It is also interesting, as one gets older, that those over 70 so often say, "My God, how fast it all went. I can't believe I'm this old now. Where did those years go?" I think people 150 or 160 will also say, "My God, where did all those years go?" Of course, if we double life expectancy, and we get everybody up to 150, 180, and if it was really terrific, then they will want more. They will say, "Why should we stop now? It's been wonderful. Let's keep going." We would have an infinite treadmill of more and more people living longer and longer, which would increase the social problems enormously.

DISCUSSION

STOCK: I don't know quite where to begin. For starters, Dr. Callahan, you seem to feel that we need to solve all the problems in advance before we can embark on a path with such profound social implications. By your logic, which is essentially that of the precautionary principle, we should have stopped medicine in the 1900s or at any time before, since the progress that made possible the extension of life expectancy, from around 45 then to 75 today, not only couldn't have been shown in advance to be benign, but also has contributed to problems from population growth to dramatic shifts in family dynamics and the role of women. By your arguments, we wouldn't want birth control; we wouldn't want telephones, computers or any new technologies. We wouldn't want to do anything that has profound effects because there is no way we can solve the problems in advance.

CALLAHAN: Would I have said the same thing 100 years ago? Absolutely not. But we have now had 100 years of technology to draw upon. We have some knowledge of what it means to society to have people live much longer lives. We have a sense of what it means to our society security system. We know what it means for the provision of health care. We know something about what it means for family life. We are not ignorant of these factors, nor could we make perfect predictions, but we could get a pretty good sense of likely possibilities on the basis of our present experience. For instance, I've become interested in universities; what happens now in universities that don't have mandatory retirement? First, some 5 to 10% of the faculty stay on beyond 70. One consequence is that often they are not very good teachers any longer and they don't work hard. They *are*, however, quite skilled at avoiding the committee assignments. But, most importantly, they block the entry of young people on to the faculty.

STOCK: The problem with your logic is that you are assuming that people are aging, that they are getting older, and their faculties are diminishing. But you can't use such an example as a way of attacking the possibility of extending our vitality rather than our decrepitude.

CALLAHAN: No, no—I'm not saying their faculties are diminished. They simply don't have their earlier energy or interest. Why do we assume this is all going to radically change by virtue of anti-aging research?

STOCK: I think that if you were now physically and mentally what you were at 40 or 50, your attitudes might be somewhat different about what it's like to be a 73-year old. You even said, "I don't want to die prematurely" and yet...

CALLAHAN: I guess there's a factor that enters in that has nothing to do with physical energy—the boredom and repetition of life. I ran an organization for 27 years. I didn't get physically tired. I just got bored doing the same thing over and over. When I think of doubling life expectancy the question that arises is how you are going to deal with the problem of boredom. Do you really believe that human beings are going to find everything brand new all the time?

STOCK: Maybe you should try doing something different.

CALLAHAN: It gets very hard to do something utterly different, even if you have the physical energy to do so. I don't know many people over my age who have started doing something radically different. My mother took up painting at the age of 70, which she had always wanted to do, and she won prizes by the time she died at 86. But by and large even most people in perfectly good health, and with money, don't start on brand new careers in their later years.

STOCK: In perfectly good health, but only for a person beyond the age of 70.

CALLAHAN: No, in perfectly good health period. These people are running around. They have plenty of energy to go on cruises and play golf—they do that sort of thing very well, but they are not interested in starting new careers. When he was in his 70s, the late journalist I. F. Stone did what he always wanted to do—he learned Greek in order to read Socrates. He then wrote a book on the Socratic dialogues in his 80s. But that's pretty rare and it was much remarked upon as unusual.

STOCK: You were talking about premature death. And yet you wouldn't want to die prematurely would you?

CALLAHAN: It wouldn't be premature if I died now.

STOCK: The notion of what constitutes premature death changes as we accept longer lives. I know a man who retired at 65 and shortly thereafter found he had cancer and died. The general reaction was, "Oh, what a tragedy, just before he was going to embark on his retirement." So you may say, "Look, you've lived long enough and you could die tomorrow and it wouldn't be premature." But remember, when Social Security was set up and retirement was set at 65, the age was chosen because hardly anyone was expected to make it that far.

CALLAHAN: Here's my definition of prematurity—not dying before one has lived a life that is long enough to allow one to do most, though not necessarily all, of the things that life enables one to do. In any case, by the time I'd reached 65, I'd raised a family, I'd had a career, I'd written a lot of books, I'd given hundreds of lectures, and I'd had lots of friends. I had not been to Nepal, and could always imagine new things I'd like to do. But I've had most of the things life has to offer. You don't have to live to be 100 to do that.

STOCK: It's astonishing to me that you could believe that you have already done most of what life allows one to do. You have an imagination. Can you not see huge realms of life that remain?

CALLAHAN: I sure can't. All I can do is keep writing more of those books and that's getting a bit repetitious now. I don't see anyone else doing it either at my age. Not just me. I'm looking at my age-mates.

STOCK: There are many people who, at a later age, do not feel they have exhausted what life has to offer.

CALLAHAN: They want to play golf in Scottsdale. That's true. Somebody once said to me, "What about the people who *like* to sit on the back porch and watch the sunset?" OK, you can do that indefinitely. If that's their life, then fine. I give in.

STOCK: You said a problem with extending longevity is that it wouldn't solve any of the major problems of the world. But why should that be a requirement? There are many things going on in society that we accept even though they aren't oriented towards solving big problems. And many people would say the decay we face with aging and decrepitude *is* a big problem that they'd like to solve or at least postpone. And effective anti-aging medicine would certainly help with that.

CALLAHAN: Radically extending life expectancy would radically change the social structure of society. Therefore, if you are going to make that kind of change, particularly just to satisfy individual desires to live longer, then I must ask, "Is this going to help the rest of us with all of our other problems?" Don't change the whole society unless you can show it is going to solve some present problems. That seems to me to be a simple proposition.

STOCK: Society is going to undergo profound change whether we extend the human life span or not, considering advances like telecommunications, computers, the Internet and all the other things that are so drastically and quickly changing society. Birth control is an obvious example of something with a dramatic impact. Society is undergoing profound change and will continue to do so. We can't hope to keep it as it is.

CALLAHAN: But at what point do we want to stop some of the profound changes? One of the changes I have been fascinated with is that we are getting more and more automobiles in this world. We need a birth control pill for automobiles. I have written a paper comparing medical technology to automobiles and had a lot of fun doing it because, on the one hand, we don't seem to be able to control the cost of medical technology, and yet we can't give it up either. On the other hand, we don't know how to count the ever-rising number of automobiles, creating all kinds of environmental and social problems, but we can't give up cars either. Ought we to have more and more cars just because individuals want more and more?

STOCK: You can argue that there are negative externalities for certain kinds of activity. But you haven't made a good case that there is a negative externality for longer life. You asked, "What is good for society? If individuals gain what they want, then why is that necessarily good for society?" Who, in your view, is actually going to decide what is good for society? Clearly, you have some very clear ideas that are in opposition to what many people believe because if they get more life they will just want even more.

CALLAHAN: I'll give you an example. A lot of people don't like to be taxed, and a lot of people particularly don't like high taxes. Yet we have decided, for the good of society, that we need taxes to pay for Social Security and Medicare, and to run our police departments, for example. We thwart a lot of individual desires by having a system of taxation. But to run a society, you have to both say no to people and to require people to do what they don't want to do. There are some higher goods than what we personally want. We set speed limits—you can't drive 90 miles an hour, even though you want to, because you may hurt others.

STOCK: So you are saying that if a majority declared they weren't interested in anti-aging medicine because it would be bad for society, then this would be something we should ban.

CALLAHAN: If you have a majority in favor of something, then you could have a tyranny of the majority. They might win and I'd lose the battle. I hope there never will be a majority in favor of a doubled life expectancy.

STOCK: When you spoke about taxation, weren't you talking about majority decisions? Weren't you saying that the political process is what should decide what is best for society?

CALLAHAN: We ought to decide politically, but I would prefer to spend a lot of money on distributing AIDS drugs than spending money on anti-aging research. Is that a bad priority on my part? Millions of people are dying of AIDS.

STOCK: Why do you have a problem with those deaths, considering it's a pretty natural path?

CALLAHAN: No it's not. AIDS leads to a *premature* death, the death of people at a young age, and affects people who are responsible for the infrastructure of society. AIDS is a terrible disease and ought to be cured. I don't think cancer in 95-year-olds needs to be cured. It's a simple as that.

STOCK: Are you suggesting that there should be some age threshold above which you don't treat people, independent of what their level of vitality is?

CALLAHAN: That's a question of how much you want to spend on Medicare. How much do you want to invest in high technology medicine to keep elderly people alive? That's going to be a problem in future years with our

Medicare system. I think you will agree we are going to have to make some very difficult decisions. Right now there are a lot of new cardiac technologies coming along—most of them very expensive, and Medicare is struggling right now to decide whether or not to provide reimbursement for them.

STOCK: How to allocate public resources is a large issue, and lots of arguments are made about the best way to spend money to best serve society as a whole. But if it becomes possible to extend the human life span and to prolong our years of vitality significantly, would you argue that there should be some sort of prohibition to stop all those who are going to want it?

CALLAHAN: I would not want to prohibit the research; rather, I would want to *stigmatize* it. I want to make it look like you are being an utterly irresponsible citizen if you would dump this radical life extension on the rest of us, as if you expect your friends and neighbors to pay for your Social Security at age 125, and your Medicare at 145. I want to make it look like one of the worst things you could do to your neighbor. That's all. I wouldn't prohibit it.

STOCK: But how can you imagine it would be stigmatized if the vast majority of people would do virtually anything to have it and if it's already something that people seek?

CALLAHAN: I would lose. I probably won't succeed in stigmatizing it, but it is worth a try.

Regulatory Mechanisms Controlling Gene Expression Mediated by the Antioxidant Response Element

THOMAS W. KENSLER

Division of Toxicological Services, Department of Environmental Health Sciences, Johns Hopkins Bloomberg School of Public Health, Baltimore, Maryland 21205, USA

Inducers of phase 2 and antioxidative genes are known to enhance the detoxification of environmental carcinogens in animals, often leading to protection against neoplasia. The use of enzyme inducers such as oltipraz (a dithiolethione) and sulforaphane (an isothiocyanate) as cancer chemopreventive agents in humans is currently under clinical investigation. A common *cis*-acting sequence, the Antioxidant Response Element (ARE), is found in the promoter regions of these protective genes. Several transcription factors are known to bind to this motif, such as members of the basic leucine zipper NF-E2 (nuclear factor erythroid-derived 2) family. One such factor, Nrf2, appears critical for the regulation of inducible and/or basal expression of genes by the ARE. An actin-binding protein, Keap1 (Kelch-like ECH-associated protein1), sequesters Nrf2 in the cytoplasm by binding to its amino-terminal regulatory domain. Keap1 is a sulfhydryl-rich protein, and several cysteine residues mediate the Keap1-inducer interaction. Treatment with oltipraz or sulforaphane disrupts the interaction between Keap1 and Nrf2, allowing Nrf2 to translocate to the nucleus. In the nucleus, Nrf2 forms heterodimers with small Maffamily proteins to activate gene expression. Highlighting the importance of this signaling pathway, *Nrf2*-deficient mice are considerably more sensitive to carcinogenesis than wild-type mice, perhaps reflecting a lower constitutive expression of carcinogen detoxification enzymes. Moreover, the cancer chemopreventive efficacies of oltipraz and sulforaphane are completely lost in the knockout mice. Hepatic gene expression patterns have been examined by oligonucleotide microarray analyses in vehicle- and dithiolethione-treated wild-type and *nrf2*-deficient mice to identify genes contributing to protection against environmental carcinogenesis.

Address for correspondence: Thomas W. Krensler, Ph.D., Director, Division of Toxicological Services, Bloomberg School of Public Health, Johns Hopkins University, 615 N. Wolfe Street, Baltimore, MD 21205. Voice: 410-955-4712.

tkensler@jhuph.edu

Ann. N.Y. Acad. Sci. 1055: 219 (2005). © 2005 New York Academy of Sciences.
doi: 10.1196/annals.1323.001

Targeting Redox Signaling Pathways for Anti-Inflammatory and Anti-Ischemic Drug Discovery

GUY MILLER

Edison Pharmaceuticals, Inc., San Jose, California 95138, USA

Increasingly, we are learning that many diseases associated with an aging population have an important inflammatory component. Data in support of this are being derived from both epidemiological and prospective investigations. For example, studies have confirmed the incidental benefit of non-steroidal anti-inflammatory drugs (NSAIDs) in limiting the progression and incidence of neurodegenerative diseases. Similarly, a variety of preclinical and clinical investigations are targeting novel inflammatory pathways in disease states such as asthma, stroke, and macular degeneration. Anti-inflammatory activities of selected pharmaceuticals, in addition to their primary mechanism of action, are now known to underlie their composite efficacies (e.g., as in statins). While considerable attention is currently being paid to targeting inflammatory disease pathways, the rate of development of pre-clinical discovery tools and drug leads has not kept pace to adequately interrogate the complex myriad pathways associated with inflammatory disease. In part, this is due to limitations in biological modeling of inflammatory pathways and diseases and in the identification of prototypic anti-inflammation chemical scaffolds for drug development. Redox-signaling pathways and oxidative stress triggers are major contributory elements to inflammation and ischemic disease. Attention will be focused upon the characterization of critical elements for successful drug discovery in the area of complex multifactorial inflammatory diseases of aging.

Address for correspondence: Guy Miller, M.D., Ph.D., Edison Pharmaceuticals, 5941 Optical Court, Suite 228, San Jose, CA 95138. Voice: 408-960-2910; fax: 408-413-5300.
gmiller@edisonpharma.com

Ann. N.Y. Acad. Sci. 1055: 220 (2005). © 2005 New York Academy of Sciences.
doi: 10.1196/annals.1323.003

Mitochondrial Thioredoxin: Critical Protection for the Redox Throttle of Life

DEAN P. JONES

Department of Medicine and Clinical Biomarkers Laboratory and Center for Clinical and Molecular Nutrition, Emory University School of Medicine, Atlanta, Georgia, 30322, USA

We previously found that mitochondrial release of cytochrome c in apoptosis triggers an intracellular respiratory burst in which the mitochondrial cytochrome $bc1$ complex generates large amounts of superoxide anion. Our subsequent studies with depletion of cellular glutathione showed that controlled generation of reactive oxygen species (ROS) at this site provides molecular communication between bioenergetic function and cellular antioxidant defenses, thus establishing a key link in cell survival signaling. The redox balance can be measured *in vivo* in humans in terms of the thiol/disulfide redox state of glutathione and cysteine in blood plasma. Glutathione redox state is constant until 45–50 years and then becomes increasingly oxidized with age. In contrast, cysteine/cystine redox is more slowly oxidized throughout life. These studies suggest that the cysteine/cystine redox can function in longevity signaling by integration of dietary, environmental and genetic risk factors that determine life span. A cellular/extracellular redox cycle links this signaling to mitochondrial bioenergetics through ROS generation, thereby maintaining inter-organ homeostasis. Our recent studies show that the unique mitochondrial form of thioredoxin is critical to this mechanism. Thioredoxins have dual functions in eliminating ROS and repairing protein damage caused by ROS. Mitochondrial thioredoxin is expressed in association with respiratory activity, providing protection against oxidant-induced apoptosis. We used a novel redox Western blot to show that mitochondrial thioredoxin is more vulnerable to oxidation than is cytoplasmic thioredoxin. Further studies to examine subcellular compartmentation of redox show that redox signaling involves discrete localized signaling pathways which can be disrupted by excessive mitochondrial ROS generation. By protecting the mitochondrial machinery, mitochondrial thioredoxin thereby provides critical protection for this redox throttle of life.

Address for correspondence: Dean P. Jones, Ph.D., Director, Clinical Biomarkers Laboratory, Emory University School of Medicine, Whitehead Biomedical Research Building, Suite 205P, 615 Michael Street, Atlanta GA 30322. Voice: 404-727-7350; fax: 727-5363.
dpjones@emory.edu

Ann. N.Y. Acad. Sci. 1055: 221 (2005). © 2005 New York Academy of Sciences.
doi: 10.1196/annals.1323.006

Regulation of Aging by SIR2

LEONARD P. GUARANTE

Department of Biology, Massachusetts Institute of Technology, Cambridge, Massachusetts 02139, USA

Aging is a process that is multifactorial, because it has largely escaped the forces of selection. Survival mechanisms, in contrast, have been selected for and are relatively simple. SIR2 is one such mechanism. In yeast this gene promotes longevity in mother cells. It also allows formation of the specialized cell type, the spore. In worms SIR-2.1 also promotes longevity in adults and formation of a specialized, long-lived form, the dauer. In mammalian cells, SIRT1 promotes survival by inhibiting p53-dependent apoptosis. The NAD-dependent deacetylase activity allows the protein to interface with metabolic activity of cells and to set the pace of aging accordingly. The link between SIRT1, white fat, and calories provides a possible pathway connecting longevity to calorie restriction in mammals.[1] More information can be found at <http://web.mit.edu/biology/guarente/references/references.html>.

REFERENCE

1. PICARD, F., M. KUTEV, N. CHUNG, *et al.* 2004. Sirt1 promotes fat mobilization in white adipocytes by repressing PPARγ. Nature. doi 10.1038/nature02583.

Address for correspondence: Leonard P. Guarante, Ph.D., Novartis Professor of Biology, Department of Biology, Massachusetts Institute of Technology, 77 Massachusetts Avenue, Cambridge, MA 02139. Voice: 617-253-6965; fax 617-253-8699.
leng@mit.edu

Ann. N.Y. Acad. Sci. 1055: 222 (2005). © 2005 New York Academy of Sciences.
doi: 10.1196/annals.1323.008

Androgens in the Aging Man

WILLIAM J. BREMNER

Department of Medicine, University of Washington School of Medicine, Seattle, Washington 98195, USA

Changes in blood levels of testosterone in men as they age are characterized by gradual declines, beginning in the 30s and continuing through their lives. Blood levels of total testosterone decrease approximately 1.5% per year. Sex hormone–binding globulin increases somewhat with age (approximately 1% per year), so levels of free testosterone and "weakly bound" or "bioavailable" testosterone decline more rapidly (2.5–3.0% per year). In some series, by age 80, 50% of men have total testosterone levels in the hypogonadal range (less than 2.5 percentile), and over 80% of men have free testosterone levels in the hypogonadal category. Some aspects of aging resemble hypogonadism (e.g., decreases in muscle, bone, and sexual interest and function, and increases in fat). Studies suggest that administration of testosterone will partially reverse some of these changes. There is general agreement that it is reasonable to strongly consider testosterone replacement for frank hypogonadism in men of any age; it is less clear and requires additional study whether testosterone replacement is advisable for more modest age-associated declines in testosterone levels.

Address for correspondence: William J. Bremner, M.D., Ph.D., The Robert G. Petersdorf Professor and Chair, Department of Medicine, University of Washington School of Medicine, Seattle, Washington 98195. Voice: 206-543-3293; fax: 206-543-3497.

wbremner@u.washington.edu

Ann. N.Y. Acad. Sci. 1055: 223 (2005). © 2005 New York Academy of Sciences.

doi: 10.1196/annals.1323.012

Potential Adverse Effects of Administering Testosterone to Elderly Men

PETER J. SNYDER

Division of Endocrinology. Diabetes and Metabolism, University of Pennsylvania School of Medicine, Philadelphia, Pennsylvania, USA

Several diseases to which elderly men are prone are thought to be testosterone-dependent, which raises the concern that administration of testosterone to elderly men might exacerbate these diseases. These diseases include prostate cancer, benign prostatic hyperplasia, erythrocytosis, and, less certainly, sleep apnea. Huggins first demonstrated the testosterone-dependence of prostate cancer more than 50 years ago when he showed that castration of men who had metastatic prostate cancer lessened the metastases.[1] Current treatment of metastatic prostate cancer still employs this principle, in the form of GnRH analogues that severely lower the serum testosterone concentration and androgen receptor antagonists. White first demonstrated the testosterone-dependence of benign prostatic hyperplasia more than one hundred years ago, showing that castration improved severe urinary obstruction due to prostatic hyperplasia.[2] The current application of this principle employs blocking the conversion of testosterone to its active metabolite, 5α-dihyrotestosterone, by finasteride or dutasterid. Although several studies have been performed recently in which elderly men were given testosterone, none showed a greater occurrence of any of these conditions than occurred in placebo-treated men, however. None of these studies, however, had sufficient power to be able to draw conclusions.

REFERENCES

1. HUGGINS, C. & C.V. HODGES. 1941. Studies on prostatic cancer: I. The effect of castration, of estrogen and of androgen injection on serum phosphatases in metastatic carcinoma of the prostate. J. Urol. **168:** 9–12.
2. WHITE, J.W. 1895. The results of double castration in hypertrophy of the prostate. Ann. Surg. 22: 1–80.

Address for correspondence: Peter J. Snyder, M.D., University of Pennsylvania Division of Endocrinology, Diabetes and Metabolism, 415 Curie Boulevard, 752A Clinical Research Building, Philadelphia, PA 19104-6149. Voice: 215-898-0208; fax: 215-573-5809.
pjs@pobox.upenn.edu

Ann. N.Y. Acad. Sci. 1055: 224 (2005). © 2005 New York Academy of Sciences.
doi: 10.1196/annals.1323.015

Testosterone in Women

ADRIAN S. DOBS

Division of Endocrinology & Metabolism, Department of Medicine, Johns Hopkins University School of Medicine, Baltimore, Maryland 21205, USA

Androgen production in women is primarily derived from the adrenals and ovaries. As women age, with the decline of DHEA from the adrenal gland, there is a reduction in circulating serum androgens, particularly after the menopause. In light of the significant controversy about estrogen replacement after menopause, there is interest in the safety and efficacy of testosterone treatment in women. Research is now accumulating to suggest that testosterone replacement therapy can have several effects that may be beneficial: increased bone density, increased lean body mass, decreased fat mass, and improved sexual function and quality of life. At this time, the proposal is quite controversial and little data are available on the long-term effects. Ongoing studies are attempting to quantitate any beneficial effects, as well as side effects.

Address for correspondence: Adrian S. Dobs, M.D., Division of Endocrinology & Metabolism, Department of Medicine, Johns Hopkins University School of Medicine, 1830 Building #328, 550 North Broadway, Baltimore, MD 21205. Voice: 410-955-2130; fax: 410-955-8172.
adobs@jhu.edu

Ann. N.Y. Acad. Sci. 1055: 225 (2005). © 2005 New York Academy of Sciences.
doi: 10.1196/annals.1323.016

Estrogen: Metabolism, Actions and Effects

JAMES W. SIMPKINS

Department of Pharmacology & Neuroscience, University of North Texas Health Science Center at Fort Worth, Fort Worth, Texas 76107, USA

Estrogen has a variety of effects in the brain that indicate the need for life-long exposure to this important steroid hormone to maintain brain health. These effects include trophic actions on neurons, resulting in enhanced synaptic connections, and neuroprotective actions, serving to protect neurons during acute insults as well as more chronic neurodegenerative diseases. A large component of the neuroprotective effects of estrogens relates to their ability to be redox cycled between the parent estrogen and 10-hydroxy-quiniols, oxidized forms of estrogens that we have recently identified in brain and other tissues. This redox cycling of estrogens allows small concentrations of estrogens effectively to block extensive membrane lipid peroxidation. This novel mechanism of estrogen neuroprotection allowed us to synthesize a large number of estrogen-like compounds that maintain their ability to neuroprotect, but which do not bind to estrogen receptors. We have demonstrated a strong correlation between the antioxidant activity of these estrogen-like molecules and their neuroprotectant activity. Additionally, several of these compounds have been tested in a variety of *in vivo* models for neuronal death and been shown to be potently neuroprotective. Collectively, these results indicate that novel estrogens can be discovered that have neuroprotective activity, but which lack many of the side effects associated with chronic estrogen use. These compounds may be useful therapeutic agents.

ACKNOWLEDGMENT

This work was supported by National Institute on Aging (NIH) Grants AG10485 and AG22550 and by MitoKor, Inc.

Address for correspondence: James W. Simpkins, Ph.D., Department of Pharmacology & Neuroscience, University of North Texas Health Science Center at Fort Worth, 3500 Camp Bowie Blvd., Fort Worth, TX 76107-2699. Voice: 817-735-2056; fax: 817-735-2091.
jsimpkin@hsc.unt.edu

Ann. N.Y. Acad. Sci. 1055: 226 (2005). © 2005 New York Academy of Sciences.
doi: 10.1196/annals.1323.017

Estrogen and the Heart: Choices for Prevention of Coronary Vascular Disease

DAVID M. HERRINGTON

Section on Cardiology, Department of Internal Medicine, Wake Forest University School of Medicine, Winston-Salem, North Carolina, USA

Recent unexpected negative results from randomized clinical trials, including the Women's Health Initiative, have completely transformed our understanding of the effect of hormone replacement therapy (HRT) on CVD risk from one of presumed benefit to one of possible harm. This surprising turn of events has made it clear that the effects of HRT on vascular health are far more complex than initially assumed and urgently in need of additional study. Understanding how it is that estrogen, which has such favorable effects on intermediate pathways such as lipid metabolism and endothelial function, could nonetheless increase risk for CHD events would undoubtedly shed new light on the pathogenesis of atherosclerosis and provide fundamentally important additional information concerning estrogen biology. New evidence from the ERA (Estrogen Replacement and Atherosclerosis) and HERS (Heart and Estrogen/Progestin Replacement Study) trials suggests that genetic variability in the estrogen receptor may account for some of the recent unexpected findings.

Address for correspondence: David M. Herrington, M.D., Department of Internal Medicine - Cardiology, Medical Center Blvd., Winston-Salem, NC 27157. Voice: 336-716-4950; fax: 336-716-9188.
dherring@wfubmc.edu

Ann. N.Y. Acad. Sci. 1055: 227 (2005). © 2005 New York Academy of Sciences.
doi: 10.1196/annals.1323.019

Estrogen, Cognition, and Dementia

SANJAY ASTHANA

Section of Geriatrics and Gerontology, Department of Medicine, University of Wisconsin School of Medicine, Madison, Wisconsin 53705, USA

Estrogen is a complex gonadal hormone that exerts numerous neurobehavioral and biological effects on the brain. Among others, these effects include the ability of estrogen to favorably modulate mechanisms underlying cognitive function and its potential to exhibit neuroprotective properties. Additionally, estrogen can favorably alter a number of neurobiological processes underlying the pathobiology of Alzheimer's disease (AD). Thus, it has been hypothesized that administration of estrogen could enhance cognition and reduce risk of postmenopausal Alzheimer's disease. Although not universally confirmed, findings from a number of randomized clinical studies indicate that administration of estrogen can enhance cognitive function of healthy older women. Further, results from numerous epidemiological studies strongly suggest that estrogen therapy can significantly reduce risk of Alzheimer's disease for postmenopausal women. However, recent findings from the Women's Health Initiative (WHI) and Women's Health Initiative Memory Study (WHIMS) raise serious concerns about the safety and feasibility of prolonged therapy with opposed oral conjugated estrogen (i.e., Prempro) and its potential to reduce risk for Alzheimer's disease.

Address for correspondence: Sanjay Asthana, M.D., Department of Geriatrics and Gerontology, University of Wisconsin Medical School, 2870 University Avenue, Suite 106, Madison, WI 53705. Voice: 608-262-8597; fax: 608-263-7645.
sa@medicine.wisc.edu

Ann. N.Y. Acad. Sci. 1055: 228 (2005). © 2005 New York Academy of Sciences.
doi: 10.1196/annals.1323.020

Use of Growth Hormone for Prevention of Effects of Aging

S. MITCHELL HARMAN

Kronos Longevity Research Institute, Phoenix, Arizona, USA

Decreases in growth hormone (GH) and circulating insulin-like growth factor-I (IGF-I), estrogen deficiency in women, and diminished levels of testosterone in men, as well as loss of lean body mass (LBM), increased body fat, and other changes consistent with hormone deficiencies occur during human aging. Treatment of non-elderly GH-deficient adults with recombinant human GH (rhGH) improves body composition, muscle strength, physical function, and bone density and appears to reduce blood cholesterol and the risk of cardiovascular disease. However, GH use is often accompanied by adverse effects, such as carpal tunnel syndrome, fluid retention with peripheral edema, joint pain and swelling, gynecomastia, glucose intolerance, and, possibly, an increased risk of cancer. Reports that rhGH increases LBM and reduces body fat in elderly men have led to public interest in using rhGH to delay effects of aging. However, to date, clinically significant functional benefits have not been demonstrated in controlled trials in older persons without pituitary disease. Moreover, marketing of rhGH and other hormone supplements by "anti-aging medicine" doctors largely ignores the extent to which the above-noted adverse effects occur in the elderly. Finally, the oft-repeated claim that GH treatment prolongs youth and extends life is unsupported by any human or animal research trials. Thus, caution is warranted with regard to age-related hormone interventions. Until more research using a variety of treatment paradigms has better defined risk/benefit ratios, treatment of elderly men and women with rhGH should be confined to properly controlled research studies.[1–4]

Competing interests statement: The author declares that he has no competing interests.

Address for correspondence: S. Mitchell Harman, M.D., Ph.D., KLRI, 2222 E. Highland Avenue, Suite 220, Phoenix, AZ 85016. Voice: 866-878-1221;fax: 602-778-7490.
mitchell.harman@kronosinstitute.org

Ann. N.Y. Acad. Sci. 1055: 229–230 (2005). © 2005 New York Academy of Sciences.
doi: 10.1196/annals.1323.026

REFERENCES

1. CARROLL, P.V., E.R. CHRIST, B.A. BENGTSSON, *et al.* 1998. Growth hormone deficiency in adulthood and the effects of growth hormone replacement: a review. Growth Hormone Research Society Scientific Committee. J. Clin. Endocrinol. Metab. **83:** 382–395.
2. ABS, R., B.A. BENGTSSON, E. HERNBERG-STAHL, *et al.* 1999. GH replacement in 1034 growth hormone deficient hypopituitary adults: demographic and clinical characteristics, dosing and safety. Clin. Endocrinol. (Oxf.) **50:** 703–713.
3. RUDMAN, D., A.G. FELLER, H.S. NAGRAJ, *et al.* 1990. Effects of human growth hormone in men over 60 years old. N. Engl. J. Med. **323:** 1–6.
4. BLACKMAN, M.R., J.D. SORKIN, T. MUNZER, *et al.* 2002. Growth hormone and sex steroid administration in healthy aged women and men: a randomized clinical trial. **288:** 2282–2292.

Cardiovascular Risk Assessment

HARVEY S. HECHT

Department of Interventional Cardiology, Lenox Hill Hospital,
New York, New York 10021

Conventional risk assessment is based upon formulas such as the Framingham Risk Score that incorporate the standard risk factors of hypertension, diabetes, smoking, age, sex, family history, and cholesterol into an estimate of cardiac event likelihood for a 10-year period. Treatment recommendations are then based upon the calculated risk. The assumptions are:

(1) that the formula accurately predicts risk;

(2) that risk in individual patients is similar to that of the "average" patient in large series of patients; and

(3) that "normal" lipid values apply equally to all patients.

In reality, these assumptions are not valid. Using the Framingham Risk Score-guided NCEP guidelines, only 25% of young patients (men < 55 years, women < 65 years) presenting with a myocardial infarction as the first symptom would be considered of sufficiently high risk before the event to warrant statin therapy; 70% were in the lowest-risk categories.

TABLE 1

CAC Score/%	Framingham Risk Group Equivalent	LDL Goal	ASA
0 0–1	Risk factors: Framingham risk assessment not required	<190	No
1–10 and <75th %ile	Low risk: (1–10% Framingham 10-year risk)	<160	No
11–100 and <75th %ile	Intermediate risk: (11–20% Framingham 10-year risk)	<130	Yes
>100 or >75th %ile	High risk; CAD risk equivalent (> 20% Framingham 10-year risk)	<100	Yes
>400 or >90th %ile	Highest risk (50–70% Framingham 10-year risk)	<100	Yes

NOTE: Statin initiated even if baseline LDL <100. ACE inhibitors and beta blockers advisable.

Address for correspondence: Dr. Harvey Hecht, Chief of Cardiovascular Computed Tomography, Department of Interventional Cardiology, Lenox Hill Hospital, 9th floor, 130 E. 77th St., New York, NY, 10021. Voice: 212-434-2606; fax: 212-434-2205.
hhecht@aol.com

Ann. N.Y. Acad. Sci. 1055: 231–232 (2005). © 2005 New York Academy of Sciences.
doi: 10.1196/annals.1323.023

Surrogate markers of atherosclerosis offer a more attractive alternative since they reflect the cumulative effect of an individual's life on the vasculature. Electron Beam Tomography (EBT) measurement of calcified coronary plaque is the most powerful surrogate marker. Several studies have demonstrated significant superiority to the Framingham Risk Score. The test is best suited for risk assessment in the conventional intermediate-risk population, although patients perceived to be at low and high risk may also benefit. Based upon the coronary calcium scores, treatment algorithms are on the previous page in TABLE 1.

Serial calcified plaque imaging also holds great promise for the assessment of the effects of treatment.

Index of Contributors

Asthana, S., 228

Bahar, R., 35–47
Bremner, W.J., 223
Brinton, E.A., 159–178
Busuttil, R.A., 35–47

Callahan, D., 207–218
Cantor, C.R., 48–57, 58–64
Chowdhury, K., 136–158
Cutler, R.G., ix–x , 58–64, 93–135,
    136–158

Dobs, A.S., 225
Dollé, M.E.T., 35–47

Guarante, L.P., 58–64, 222

Harman, S.M., 229–230
Hecht, H.S., 231–232
Herrington, D.M., 227
Heward, C., 136–158

Jones, D.P., 58–64, 221

Kaput, J., 64–79
Kensler, T.W., 58–64, 219

Lands, W.E.M., 179–192

Martin, G.M., 26–34, 58–64
Masutani, H., 1–12
Miller, G., 220
Moffat, S.D., 80–92

Naftolin, F., 58–64
Nakamura, H., 1–12

Perls, T., 13–25
Plummer, J., 136–158

Simpkins, J.W., 226
Snyder, P.J., 224
Stewart, K.J., 193–206
Stock, G.B., 207–218

Vijg, J., 35–47

Yodoi, J., 1–12
Yoshida, T., 1–12